W9-BXG-141

TO HEAL THE SICK

by Charles and Frances Hunter

Published by Hunter Books
City of Light
201 McClellan Road
Kingwood, Texas 77339, U.S.A.

BOOKS BY CHARLES 💕 FRANCES HUNTER

A CONFESSION A DAY KEEPS THE DEVIL AWAY
ANGELS ON ASSIGNMENT
BORN AGAIN! WHAT DO YOU MEAN?
COME ALIVE
DELIGHTFULLY CHARISMATIC Christian Walk Seminar
    Manual
DEVIL, YOU CAN'T STEAL WHAT'S MINE
DON'T LIMIT GOD
DON'T PANIC ... PRAY!
FOLLOW ME
GOD IS FABULOUS
GOD'S ANSWER TO FAT ... LOØSE IT!
GOD'S BIG "IF"
GOD'S CONDITIONS FOR PROSPERITY
HOT LINE TO HEAVEN
HOW TO DEVELOP YOUR FAITH
HOW TO FIND GOD'S WILL FOR YOUR LIFE
HOW TO HAVE FREEDOM FROM FEAR
HOW TO MAKE YOUR MARRIAGE EXCITING
IMPOSSIBLE MIRACLES
IN JESUS' NAME!
INVEST YOUR LIFE IN GOD
IT'S SO SIMPLE (formerly HANG LOOSE WITH JESUS)
JOY, JOY, JOY!
LET'S GO WITNESSING (formerly GO, MAN! GO)
MEMORIZING MADE EASY
MY LOVE AFFAIR WITH CHARLES
NUGGETS OF TRUTH
P.T.L.A. (Praise the Lord, Anyway!)
SIMPLE AS A, B, C.
SINCE JESUS PASSED BY
SHOUT THE WORD
the fabulous SKINNIE MINNIE RECIPE BOOK
SUPERNATURAL HORIZONS (from Glory to Glory)
THE DEVIL WANTS YOUR MIND
THE TWO SIDES OF A COIN
THIS WAY UP!
TO HEAL THE SICK
WHY SHOULD "I" SPEAK IN TONGUES???

Scripture quotations are taken from:
The Authorized King James Version (KJV)
The Living Bible, Paraphrased (TLB), © *1971 by Tyndale
    House Publishers, Wheaton, Illinois.*
The Amplified Old Testament (Amp.), © *1965 by Zondervan
    Publishing*
The Amplified New Testament (Amp.), © *The Lockman
    Foundation 1954, 1958.*
All references not specified are from The Authorized King James Version.
Quotation from THE FOURTH DIMENSION, © *1979 by Paul Yonggi Cho,
    reprinted with permission by Logos International, Plainfield, New Jersey 07060.*

ISBN 0-917726-40-5

TABLE OF CONTENTS

CHAPTER	TITLE	PAGE

1. DOUBLE VISION FOR A SINGLE MISSION 5
2. THE BIG BREAKTHROUGH.................... 17
3. LAYING ON OF HANDS...................... 22
4. LAYING ON OF HANDS — PLUS............... 38
5. LET THE SICK LAY HANDS ON YOU 50
6. TALK TO A MOUNTAIN 57
7. WHAT YOU SEE IS WHAT YOU GET........... 72
8. SOME CONDITIONS FOR HEALING 93
9. ANOINTING WITH OIL 103
10. HEALING THROUGH INTER-
CESSORY PRAYER 108
11. HEALING THROUGH USE OF
PRAYER CLOTHS.............................. 111
12. OTHER WAYS TO HEAL THE SICK 115
13. WHAT IF I DON'T GET HEALED............... 127
14. BEING SENSITIVE TO THE HOLY SPIRIT...... 130
15. CASTING OUT DEVILS 135
16. THE GIFT OF FAITH 170
17. CREATIVE MIRACLES 184
18. GROWING OUT ARMS AND LEGS 197
19. GO INTO ALL THE WORLD ...
HEAL THE SICK 210

For information about the City of Light School of Ministry, Video Bible School, audio or video teaching tapes or seminar tapes, write to:

HUNTER BOOKS
City of Light
201 McClellan Road
Kingwood, Texas 77339

In the event your Christian Bookstore does not have any of the books written by Charles and Frances Hunter, please write for price list or order from Hunter Books.

CHAPTER 1
DOUBLE VISION FOR A SINGLE MISSION

By Charles and Frances

In June of 1980, God gave us a vision of the world with silver and gold bands covering the entire globe — but not in the orderly sense you would expect to see them. These bands were spilling all over the world like melted silver and gold rivulets and running into all sorts of odd little places — mountains and valleys alike. There was no obvious plan of any kind represented by these silver and gold rivulets — they went hither and thither all over the place. Sometimes they were wide, and sometimes they were super skinny. In some places it looked like a big blob of melted silver and gold had fallen, but there was no pattern of any kind! Then we saw students begin to rise up and stand on these melted silver and gold bands.

We began to ponder on this, because in the beginning it seemed to us like nothing but a huge hodgepodge, but slowly God began to reveal what this vision meant, and how it applied to our ministry.

The more we examined this divine vision, the more we began to understand that God was telling us to take the total message of salvation, which includes healing, to the entire world, by letting the masses learn how to operate in the supernatural and heal the sick.

Our hearts began to sing as God continued the revelation of what he wanted us to do. First, he directed us to teach on the subject of HOW TO HEAL THE SICK. We had seen students from the City of Light School of Ministry standing on the silver and gold bands, and thought momentarily that they were going to go to all parts of the world to teach the nationals how to heal the sick. Somehow this understanding did not give us total assurance that this was actually what the vision meant. We continued to think more about the vision.

Then the picture expanded even more, and we saw the video schools going into ALL the world — into the small places where evangelists never go, to teach all the people in the remotest places of the world how to lay hands on the sick and heal them. The students who learned from these video tapes would then go out and preach the gospel to the poor, heal the brokenhearted, preach deliverance to the captives and recovering of sight to the blind, and set at liberty those who are bruised.

For the first time, we plainly saw the identity of the students standing on the bands! We had seen students of all nationalities, but had thought they would be coming to the school here in Texas. Then we realized they were the ones we might not ever meet, the ones who might only see us through video tapes, but the ones who had received the message of how to heal the sick and had gone out to stretch forth their hands to the sick!

This is God's timing for another great move of his Spirit as the masses are being trained to go out and minister on a one-to-one basis. Bible colleges and schools of ministry have sprung up all over as a hungry world says, "Teach us how to operate in the supernatural the way the original disciples did!"

There is such a hungering among God's people to learn more about the things of God that we believe in a few years there will not be enough schools to fill the need, and the people will have to be put on a wait-list to get into the schools that are already in operation. What a thrilling thought, and what a thrilling time to be alive!

We were confident that God had opened our spirits to a dynamic, far-reaching mission of teaching the masses how simple it is to become a miracle-working disciple like those in the book of Acts.

The Monday after we finished teaching on Friday, God supernaturally sent a missionary to our school, who knew nothing about our video tape ministry, and we gave him fourteen hours of teaching on how to heal the sick.

On Tuesday, God sent another missionary! We gave him a complete set of teaching tapes as well. He had a video player in Africa, but he desperately needed tapes. He called us within two weeks and reported that he had rented a building in Tanzania (formerly Tanganyika), which would hold about three hundred people, and after inserting one small ad in the newspaper, he had turn-away crowds to see the teaching. Great numbers were healed as they watched these tapes, and eighteen were saved and baptized in water the following Sunday!

In just two or three months, video schools have started among the Catholic charismatics in Lima, Peru, and other schools are in Bolivia, the Philippines, three other countries in Africa and requests are coming in from all over the world for this particular series of tapes containing the "how to's" of healing!

As we held a Healing Seminar in Kansas shortly after this, Pastor Fred Kirkpatrick told us of a prophecy about the end times which literally exploded our faith as a confirmation of the part this teaching will play in what we believe to be the end of the end times before Jesus comes for those who love and obey him.

Our book was ready for the typesetter with the exception of the Introduction, when we contacted the

publisher of a book entitled PERTINENT PROPH-
ECIES I by John M. and Dorothea M. Gardner, and
received permission to reprint the following prophecy,
given by Tommy Hicks, noted evangelist, in 1961.

VISION OF THE BODY OF CHRIST
AND THE END-TIME MINISTRIES

*My message begins July 25, about 2:30 in the morn-
ing at Winnipeg, Canada. I had hardly fallen asleep
when the vision and the revelation that God gave me came
before me. The vision came three times, exactly in detail,
the morning of July 25, 1961. I was so stirred and so
moved by the revelation that this has changed my complete outlook upon the body of Christ, and upon the end-
time ministries.*

*The greatest thing that the church of Jesus Christ has
ever been given lies straight ahead. It is so hard to help
men and women to realize and understand the thing that
God is trying to give to his people in the end times.*

*I received a letter several weeks ago from one of our
native evangelists down in Africa, down in Nairobi. This
man and his wife were on their way to Tanganyika. They
could neither read nor could they write, but we had been
supporting them for over two years. As they entered into
the territory of Tanganyika, they came across a small
village. The entire village was evacuating because of a
plague that had hit the village. He came across natives
that were weeping, and he asked them what was wrong.*

*They told him of their mother and father who had
suddenly died, and they had been dead for three days.
They had to leave. They were afraid to go in; they were
leaving them in the cottage. He turned and asked them
where they were. They pointed to the hut and he asked
them to go with him, but they refused. They were afraid to
go.*

The native and his wife went to this little cottage and

entered in where the man and woman had been dead for three days. He simply stretched forth his hand in the name of the Lord Jesus Christ, and spoke the man's name and the woman's name and said, "In the name of the Lord Jesus Christ, I command life to come back to your bodies." Instantaneously these two heathen people who had never known Jesus Christ as their Savior sat up and immediately began to praise God. The spirit and the power of God came into the life of those people.

To us that may seem strange and a phenomenon, but that is the beginning of these end-time ministries. God is going to take the do-nothings, the nobodies, the unheard-of, the no-accounts. He is going to take every man and every woman and he is going to give to them this outpouring of the Spirit of God.

In the book of Acts we read that "In the last days," God said, "I will pour out my Spirit upon all flesh." I wonder if we realized what he meant when God said, "I will pour out my Spirit upon all flesh." I do not think I fully realize nor could I understand the fullness of it, and then I read from the book of Joel: "Be glad then, ye children of Zion, and rejoice in the Lord your God: for he hath given you the former rain moderately, and he will cause to come down for you the rain, the former rain, and the latter rain ___" (Joel 2:23). It is not only going to be the rain, the former rain and the latter rain, but he is going to give to his people in these last days a double portion of the power of God!

As the vision appeared to me after I was asleep, I suddenly found myself in a great high distance. Where I was, I do not know. But I was looking down upon the earth. Suddenly the whole earth came into my view. Every nation, every kindred, every tongue came before my sight from the east and the west, the north and the south. I recognized every country and many cities that I had been in, and I was almost in fear and trembling as I beheld the great sight before me: and at that moment when the world came into view, it began to lightning and thunder.

As the lightning flashed over the face of the earth, my eyes went downward and I was facing the north. Suddenly I beheld what looked like a great giant, and as I stared and looked at it, I was almost bewildered by the sight. It was so gigantic and so great. His feet seemed to reach to the north pole and his head to the south. Its arms were stretched from sea to sea. I could not even begin to understand whether this be a mountain or this be a giant, but as I watched, I suddenly beheld a great giant. I could see his head was struggling for life. He wanted to live, but his body was covered with debris from head to foot, and at times this great giant would move his body and act as though it would even raise up at times. And when it did, thousands of little creatures seemed to run away. Hideous creatures would run away from this giant, and when he would become calm, they would come back.

All of a sudden this great giant lifted his hand toward the heaven, and then it lifted its other hand, and when it did, these creatures by the thousands seemed to flee away from this giant and go into the darkness of the night.

Slowly this great giant began to rise and as he did, his head and hands went into the clouds. As he rose to his feet he seemed to have cleansed himself from the debris and filth that was upon him, and he began to raise his hands into the heavens as though praising the Lord, and as he raised his hands, they went even unto the clouds.

Suddenly, every cloud became silver, the most beautiful silver I have ever known. As I watched this phenomenon it was so great I could not even begin to understand what it all meant. I was so stirred as I watched it, and I cried unto the Lord and I said, "Oh, Lord, what is the meaning of this," and I felt as if I was actually in the Spirit and I could feel the presence of the Lord even as I was asleep.

And from those clouds suddenly there came great

drops of liquid light raining down upon this mighty giant, and slowly, slowly, this giant began to melt, began to sink itself in the very earth itself, and as he melted, his whole form seemed to have melted upon the face of the earth, and this great rain began to come down. Liquid drops of light began to flood the very earth itself and as I watched this giant that seemed to melt, suddenly it became millions of people over the face of the earth. As I beheld the sight before me, people stood up all over the world! They were lifting their hands and they were praising the Lord.

At that very moment there came a great thunder that seemed to roar from the heavens. I turned my eyes toward the heavens and suddenly I saw a figure in white, in glistening white — the most glorious thing that I have ever seen in my entire life. I did not see the face, but somehow I knew it was the Lord Jesus Christ, and he stretched forth his hand, and as he did, he would stretch it forth to one, and to another, and to another. And as he stretched forth his hand upon the nations and the people of the world —men and women — as he pointed toward them, this liquid light seemed to flow from his hands into them, and a mighty anointing of God came upon them, and those people began to go forth in the name of the Lord.

I do not know how long I watched it. It seemed it went into days and weeks and months. And I beheld this Christ as he continued to stretch forth his hand; but there was a tragedy. There were many people as he stretched forth his hand that refused the anointing of God and the call of God. I saw men and women that I knew. People that I felt would certainly receive the call of God. But as he stretched forth his hand toward this one and toward that one, they simply bowed their head and began to back away. And each of those that seemed to bow down and back away, seemed to go into darkness. Blackness seemed to swallow them everywhere.

I was bewildered as I watched it, but these people that

he had anointed, hundreds of thousands of people all over the world, in Africa, England, Russia, China, America, all over the world, the anointing of God was upon these people as they went forward in the name of the Lord. I saw these men and women as they went forth. They were ditch diggers, they were washerwomen, they were rich men, they were poor men. I saw people who were bound with paralysis and sickness and blindness and deafness. As the Lord stretched forth to give them this anointing, they became well, they became healed, and they went forth!

And this is the miracle of it — this is the glorious miracle of it — those people would stretch forth their hands exactly as the Lord did, and it seemed as if there was this same liquid fire in their hands. As they stretched forth their hands they said, "According to my word, be thou made whole."

As these people continued in this mighty end-time ministry, I did not fully realize what it was, and I looked to the Lord and said, "What is the meaning of this?" And he said, "This is that which I will do in the last days. I will restore all that the cankerworm, the palmerworm, the caterpillar — I will restore all that they have destroyed. This, my people, in the end times will go forth. As a mighty army shall they sweep over the face of the earth."

As I was at this great height, I could behold the whole world. I watched these people as they were going to and fro over the face of the earth. Suddenly there was a man in Africa and in a moment he was transported by the Spirit of God, and perhaps he was in Russia, or China or America or some other place, and vice versa. All over the world these people went, and they came through fire, and through pestilence, and through famine. Neither fire nor persecution, nothing seemed to stop them.

Angry mobs came to them with swords and with guns. And like Jesus, they passed through the multitudes and they could not find them, but they went forth in the name of the Lord, and everywhere they stretched forth their hands, the sick were healed, the blind eyes were opened. There was not a long prayer, and after I had reviewed the vision many times in my mind, and I thought about it many times, I realized that I never saw a church, and I never saw or heard a denomination, but these people were going in the name of the Lord of Hosts. Hallelujah!

As they marched forth in everything they did as the ministry of Christ in the end times, these people were ministering to the multitudes over the face of the earth. Tens of thousands, even millions seemed to come to the Lord Jesus Christ as these people stood forth and gave the message of the kingdom, of the coming kingdom, in this last hour. It was so glorious, but it seems as though there were those that rebelled, and they would become angry and they tried to attack those workers that were giving the message.

God is going to give to the world a demonstration in this last hour as the world has never known. These men and women are of all walks of life, degrees will mean nothing. I saw these workers as they were going over the face of the earth. When one would stumble and fall, another would come and pick him up. There were no "big I" and "little you," but every mountain was brought low and every valley was exalted, and they seemed to have one thing in common — there was a divine love, a divine love that seemed to flow forth from these people as they worked together, and as they lived together. It was the most glorious sight that I have ever known. Jesus Christ was the theme of their life. They continued and it seemed the days went by as I stood and beheld this sight. I could only cry, and sometimes I laughed. It was so wonderful as these people went throughout the face of the whole earth, bringing forth in this last end time.

As I watched from the very heaven itself, there were times when great deluges of this liquid light seemed to fall

*upon great congregations, and that congregation would
lift their hands and seemingly praise God for hours and
even days as the Spirit of God came upon them. God said,
"I will pour my Spirit upon all flesh," and that is exactly
this thing. And to every man and every woman that
received this power, and the anointing of God, the miracles of God, there was no ending to it.*

*We have talked about miracles. We have talked about
signs and wonders, but I could not help but weep as I
read again this morning, at 4 o'clock this morning the
letter from our native workers. This is only the evidence of
the beginning for one man, a "do-nothing, an unheard-of,"
who would go and stretch forth his hand and say, "In the
name of the Lord Jesus Christ, I command life to flow
into your body." I dropped to my knees and began to pray
again, and I said, "Lord, I know that this thing is coming
to pass, and I believe it's coming soon!"*

*And then again, as these people were going about the
face of the earth, a great persecution seemed to come from
every angle.*

*Suddenly there was another great clap of thunder,
that seemed to resound around the world, and I heard
again the voice, the voice that seemed to speak, "Now this
is my people. This is my beloved bride," and when the
voice spoke, I looked upon the earth and I could see the
lakes and the mountains. The graves were opened and
people from all over the world, the saints of all ages,
seemed to be rising. And as they rose from the grave,
suddenly all these people came from every direction.
From the east and the west, from the north and the south,
and they seemed to be forming again this gigantic body.
As the dead in Christ seemed to be rising first, I could
hardly comprehend it. It was so marvelous. It was so far
beyond anything I could ever dream or think of.*

*But as this body suddenly began to form, and take
shape again, it took shape again in the form of this
mighty giant, but this time it was different. It was arrayed*

in the most beautiful gorgeous white. Its garments were without spot or wrinkle as its body began to form, and the people of all ages seemed to be gathered into this body, and slowly, slowly, as it began to form up into the very heavens, suddenly from the heavens above, the Lord Jesus came, and became the head, and I heard another clap of thunder that said, "This is my beloved bride for whom I have waited. She will come forth even tried by fire. This is she that I have loved from the beginning of time."

As I watched, my eyes suddenly turned to the far north, and I saw seemingly destruction: men and women in anguish and crying out, and buildings in destruction.

Then I heard again, the fourth voice that said, "Now is My wrath being poured out upon the face of the earth." From the ends of the whole world, the wrath of God seemed to be poured out and it seemed that there were great vials of God's wrath being poured out upon the face of the earth. I can remember it as though it happened a moment ago. I shook and trembled as I beheld the awful sight of seeing the cities, and whole nations going down into destruction.

I could hear the weeping and wailing. I could hear people crying. They seemed to cry as they went into caves, but the caves in the mountains opened up.

They leaped into water, but the water would not drown them. There was nothing that could destroy them. They were wanting to take their lives, but they could not.

Then again I turned my eyes to this glorious sight, this body arrayed in beautiful white, shining garments. Slowly, slowly, it began to lift from the earth, and as it did, I awoke. What a sight I had beheld! I had seen the end-time ministries — the last hour. Again on July 27, at 2:30 in the morning, the same revelation, the same vision came again exactly as it did before.

My life has been changed as I realized that we are living in that end time, for all over the world God is anointing men and women with this ministry. It will not be doctrine. It will not be a churchianity. It is going to be Jesus Christ. They will give forth the word of the Lord, and are going to say, "I heard it so many times in the vision and according to my word it shall be done."

Oh, my people, listen to me. According to my word, it shall be done. We are going to be clothed with power and anointing from God. We won't have to preach sermons, we won't have to have persons heckle us in public. We won't have to depend on man, nor will we be denomination echoes, but we will have the power of the living God. We will fear no man, but will go in the name of the Lord of Hosts!

Can you see what we see in these two visions given twenty years apart?

CHAPTER 2
THE BIG BREAKTHROUGH

By Charles and Frances

We have been assigned and commissioned to take the gospel to all the world around us, and the only way we will be able to accomplish this is with miracles just like Jesus did!

"Jesus' disciples saw him do many other miracles besides the ones told about in this book, but these are recorded SO THAT YOU WILL BELIEVE THAT HE IS THE MESSIAH, THE SON OF GOD, AND IN BELIEVING IN HIM YOU WILL HAVE LIFE" (John 20:30,31 TLB).

We are in the very end of this age, and there is an urgency in the entire body of Christ to prepare the world for the soon-coming return of Jesus! We must reach every kindred and every tribe and every tongue with the supernatural.

How can this be done? By believing that THE SUPERNATURAL CAN BE TAUGHT! We feel in our spirits that the masses of ordinary people around the world will suddenly arise to the supernatural move of the Holy Spirit and will be healing the sick, casting out devils, and presenting a living, vital Jesus to the multitudes.

This will not be limited to the ordained ministers of the gospel, but will include the multitudes. God has anointed us and directed us to present the simple ways of healing the sick that he has been teaching us for the past few years. They have worked for us and multiplied thousands have been healed. We have taught others how to heal the sick and cast out devils, and it has worked for them. And it will for you.

Now God has told us to present this teaching throughout the world! Blind eyes are going to be opened through this book — spiritual eyes that have been clouded with tradition are going to find the scales falling off as they receive new insight concerning the healing power of God. God never intended for healing to be complicated. He made it very simple, but man tends to make it difficult. Jesus, the Great Physician, gave us the earthly healing job and said that those who believe shall lay hands on the sick and they shall recover (Mark 16:18).

Is it really God's will for people to be healed? Let's take a look:

"Large crowds followed Jesus as he came down the hillside. Look! A leper is approaching. He kneels before him, worshiping. 'Sir,' the leper pleads, 'if you want to, you can heal me.' Jesus touches the man. 'I want to,' he says, 'Be healed.' And instantly the leprosy disappears" (Matthew 8:1-3 TLB).

Yes, IT IS GOD'S WILL FOR YOU TO BE HEALED! You do not bring glory to God by walking around sick, saying, "I am being sick for the glory of God." Sickness does not bring glory to God — healing and health bring glory to God! When the leper asked Jesus to heal him, he said, "Sir, if you WANT to, you can heal me."

What was Jesus' response?

"I WANT to," Jesus said, "Be healed!"

Does Jesus want to heal you? What did he say to the leper? He said, "I WANT TO!" He says exactly the same thing to you today!

In the King James Version, this passage reads:

"And, behold, there came a leper and worshipped him, saying, Lord, if thou wilt, thou canst make me clean. And Jesus put forth his hand, and touched him, saying, I will; be thou clean. And immediately his leprosy was cleansed."

Hebrews 13:8 tells us that Jesus Christ is *"the same yesterday, and to day, and for ever."* Is it God's will to heal? In one translation, Jesus says, "I want to." In the other, he says, "I will." Neither one is negative, both say YES!

Is it really God's will for us to heal the sick? Let's take a look, because it often shocks people when you say THEY should heal the sick. The very first "religious" thought that comes to mind is that saying YOU do the healing doesn't glorify God and Jesus. Jesus very plainly told us in the great commission to lay hands on the sick, and then he simply stated they would recover. The Living Bible even makes it simpler because it says *"... and they will be able to place their hands on the sick and heal them"* (Mark 16:18).

Jesus said, *"He that believeth on me, the works that I do shall he do also; and greater works than these shall he do; because I go unto my Father"* (John 14:12).

There are many, many different ways to heal the sick. In this book we want to show you some of the surprises that God has shown us as he has taught us how easy it is to heal the sick. Healing is simple according to God's Word, but man has attempted to complicate it.

This book will teach YOU how to heal the sick in the name of Jesus, and to give GOD all the glory! You will also learn that if one method doesn't work for you, you should try another way, because if God had wanted US to heal only one particular way, he would never have had Jesus heal in so many different ways in the Bible!

A minister was watching a friend of ours operate in the gifts of the Spirit described in the twelfth chapter of

I Corinthians. He said, "Can you give me any clues which would help me to be able to operate in these gifts?"

Our friend said, "Charles and Frances Hunter taught me."

Surprised, he said, "Do you mean the supernatural can be taught?"

YES IT CAN!

This minister came to a three-day seminar where we taught on how to develop the gifts of the Spirit, went home and began to operate in all nine gifts, and to teach other ministers who were working with him. It works!

We visited an ophthalmologist who had just installed a piece of equipment with which a laser beam of light could be directed to the eye of the patient. He explained to us that if there was a tiny hole in the eye, he could direct this laser beam to the exact point of the hole, punch a button, and "zap" and the hole was sealed!

It was not the ophthalmologist who closed the hole. It was not his healing touch that accomplished the healing. It was the laser beam directed by the skillful hand of the doctor.

It was a force, an energy, a power, a laser beam that did the actual healing. But the ophthalmologist was still the doctor who applied the energy which accomplished the healing!

When the woman with an issue of blood touched the hem of Jesus' garment and was healed, Jesus said he felt healing virtue, or power, go from his body (See Mark 5:30).

Jesus was the Great Physician who applied the power of the Holy Spirit to accomplish that mighty healing, just as the ophthalmologist did.

The Holy Spirit is a thorough teacher, and he never stops teaching anyone who is willing to learn and to apply the learning for the glory of God!

To heal the sick is exciting! It is the desire of Jesus!

It is the will of God! And — for the Spirit-filled believer — it is natural!

Why don't more people heal the sick?

"My people are destroyed for lack of knowledge." (Hosea 4:6).

This book will give you the knowledge you need to heal those around you and to go around the world and heal the sick.

There is a beautiful scripture we think everyone should read. Everyone ought to know this scripture, and everyone ought to do it! It is found in the 14th chapter of Exodus, verse 15: *"Then the Lord said to Moses, quit praying and get the people moving! FORWARD, MARCH!"* (TLB).

That is what God is saying to you. "Quit praying and get moving; FORWARD, MARCH!"

Let's go through that big breakthrough and learn how to operate in the supernatural!

CHAPTER 3
LAYING ON OF HANDS

By Frances

Probably everybody who has a healing ministry has his own favorite way of healing the sick. Charles likes one way; I like another. My own favorite method is summed up in Mark 16:17,18 where Jesus says, *"And these signs shall follow them that believe; In my name shall they cast out devils; they shall speak with new tongues ... they shall lay hands on the sick, and they shall recover."* It seems to me that the simplest way to heal the sick is by the laying on of hands.

If you will notice, Jesus did not say, "Those who believe shall lay hands on the sick, they shall pray for half an hour, they shall work up tremendous emotions, they shall roll on the floor, they shall kick and holler and scream, they shall shake all over the place, and THEN the sick shall be healed." No, he very simply says, "Those who believe shall lay hands on the sick and they shall recover."

You will notice that the Bible does not leave any doubt. It does not say SOME of you, or just a FEW of you who believe; it simply says that ALL those who believe are going to be able to lay hands on the sick, and the sick ARE going to recover.

BELIEVERS are the ones who are qualified to heal the sick! But what is a believer? A believer is one who believes that Jesus is the divine Son of God and our Redeemer; but a believer is also one who believes he can cast out devils, who speaks in a spirit language; who believes he can handle Satan and his demons; who believes he can lay hands on the sick and heal them. We need to believe ALL of the way if we want ALL of that scripture to work!

You have to believe in divine healing if you want signs and wonders and miracles to follow your preaching of the Word.

You have to believe that healing is for TODAY, or else the sick won't recover when you lay hands on them.

You have to believe that you have been commissioned by the Lord Jesus Christ himself to cast out devils, or you will never cast them out!

The greatest ministry Charles and I have is probably in the area of healing, and the reason for this is that we have never been afraid to step out and do the things God has called us to do.

Sometimes we have experimented. While there are many ways to heal the sick listed in the Bible, there are also new avenues you can explore, where God will open a tremendous ministry.

"But," you might say, "it is not written in the Bible."

John said, *"And there are also many other things which Jesus did, the which, if they should be written every one, I suppose that even the world itself could not contain the books that should be written"* (John 21:25).

We need to understand that while we should never depart from the PRINCIPLES of the Bible, we can see many kinds of miracles which are not specifically described there. These are still scriptural, because they come under the authority of scriptures such as Mark 11:23 or Mark 16:18.

The first way Jesus healed during his earthly ministry was by touching people, or by "laying on of hands." "Touching" still works today!

One of the most unique miracles that I remember happened as I was coming down an aisle of a church. God impressed me to reach out and touch the top of a woman's head. This woman had cancer of the tongue. That one little touch, releasing the power of God, caused her to be totally healed of cancer and her tongue was completely restored!

When any Spirit-filled believer lays hands on someone, the power of God goes out of him into the other person. If you are Spirit-filled, you have in you the very same resurrection power that brought Jesus Christ out of the grave — the power of the Holy Spirit. You have that power residing in you at all times! You do not have to work up an emotion. I had no emotion except joy when I walked down that aisle, but God's resident power was working, because it is operable at ALL times whether you feel it or not!

Another time I walked down the aisle and touched a man with diabetes. He was instantly healed! I did not hear about either of these healings until years later, so I often wonder how many others have experienced divine healing through this method. In neither of these two cases did I "pray up a storm," nor work up emotions. I just simply touched them!

Touching does a lot in many areas of our lives. When Charles and I stand together, you will often see us reach out and touch each other's hand. The most wonderful service in the world can be going on but when I reach over and touch Charles' hand or he touches mine, somehow in a beautiful little way, that touch says, "I love you." He does not say a word. He just touches my hand, and it says, "I love you."

When you were a little child, did you ever fall down and skin your knee, and come running to your mother, screaming and hollering and carrying on? Probably she just loved you, but that TOUCH did something very special for you, didn't it? Even when you are not saved, there is a lot accomplished by touching in human love.

Did anyone ever pat your hand in a hospital when you were recovering from an operation? That did not say, "I hate you," did it? It said, "Everything is going to be all right!"

If you've ever been bereaved, hasn't it meant a lot when people just patted you, even if they couldn't say a word?

Even without words, that little touch says, "I understand your grief, and my heart goes out to you."

We need to realize how important our hands are in the healing ministry. We need to be aware of the importance of a touch!

Statistics show that babies who are given only a minimum amount of handling are inclined to be fretful, irritable and not as healthy as babies who are picked up and loved. Children who are loved and played with, and even just held have a much more loving disposition.

Sometimes people will say, "It is not God's will to heal." We need to remember that when people say this, they do not know the scriptures.

A good scripture to give them is Acts 10:38, where Peter told *"How God anointed Jesus of Nazareth with the Holy Ghost and with power: who went about doing good, and HEALING ALL that were oppressed of the devil; for God was with him."*

IT IS GOD'S WILL FOR ALL OF HIS CHILDREN TO BE HEALED.

God anointed Jesus. What was the purpose of that? God anointed Jesus so that Jesus would have the power to do what God wanted him to do. When God anointed him, he put his stamp of approval on him with the Holy Ghost and with power, and then, "He went about doing good, and healing all that were oppressed of the devil."

Acts 10:38 says that Jesus went about "healing all that were oppressed of the devil."

Sickness comes from the devil. God can take

sickness and make a miracle out of it, but God is not the one who sends sickness to his children who obey his commandments (Deut. 28).

I have heard people say, "God sent this sickness on me to teach me a lesson; he is teaching me something." I find it difficult to believe that, because would God give something as horrible as sickness to his children? Would you do that to your children? And think how much more God loves us than we love our earthly children! *"(And the Lord answered) Can a woman forget her nursing child, that she should not have compassion on the son of her womb? Yes, they may forget, yet will I not forget you"* (Isaiah 49:15 Amp).

I believe all sickness comes from the devil, but God can take it, turn it around and make it the greatest miracle in your life.

In my case, that is exactly what happened. I was in an automobile accident in 1964. Some young man ran into the back of my car and the blow that I suffered caused me to lose the sight of my left eye. That could have been a horrible tragedy, but instead, God turned it into the greatest thing that ever happened to me, because I found Jesus as a result! God took what the devil did and turned it around! After running from Jesus for 49 years, I finally accepted him!

God did not cause that accident to happen. God did not cause me to lose the sight of that eye; God had nothing to do with that part of it. But God did take that circumstance, and turn it into a miracle!

Another really good scripture is I John 3:8, "... *For this purpose the Son of God was manifested, that he might destroy the works of the devil."* Jesus was not sent here to create problems; he was sent to destroy the very works of the devil himself.

In Luke 4:18 Jesus proclaims, *"The Spirit of the Lord is upon me, because he hath anointed me to preach the gospel to the poor; he hath sent me to heal the broken-*

hearted, to preach deliverance to the captives, and recovering of sight to the blind, to set at liberty them that are bruised." Just like Jesus, we have been anointed to preach the gospel. Wherever we are, whether we have a healing ministry or some other ministry, we are always anointed to preach the gospel. That is a permanent anointing! You don't have to say, "Oh Lord, anoint me again." You have been anointed and appointed and that is why you can go out at all times and know that the anointing of God rests upon you. We KNOW that we have been dispatched to do the same things that Jesus Christ did when he was on this earth.

There are many examples in the book of Mark of how Jesus healed people. Read Mark, and then read all of the gospels, searching for just one thing: HOW DID JESUS HEAL THE SICK?

Mark 1:40-42 tells how Jesus simply "touched" the leper. He just laid hands on him, and he was healed.

Mark 5:35-40 says: "*While he yet spake, there came from the ruler of the synagogue's house certain which said, Thy daughter is dead: why troublest thou the Master any further? As soon as Jesus heard the word that was spoken, he saith unto the ruler of the synagogue, Be not afraid, only believe.*" Believing is so important! "*And he suffered no man to follow him, save Peter, and James, and John the brother of James. And he cometh to the house of the ruler of the synagogue, and seeth the tumult, and them that wept and wailed greatly. And when he was come in, he saith unto them, Why make ye this ado, and weep? the damsel is not dead, but sleepeth. And they laughed him to scorn.*"

You will notice he got the unbelievers out of the room. (Unbelief can stop healing!) Mark tells us, "*He taketh the father and the mother of the damsel, and them that were with him, and entereth in where the damsel was lying. And he took the damsel by the hand, and said unto her, Talitha cumi; which is, being interpreted, Damsel, I say unto thee, arise. And straightway the damsel arose, and walked; for she was of the age of twelve years. And they were astonished with a great astonishment."* Jesus TOUCHED the damsel's hand. At the very moment Jesus TOUCHED her hand, life came back into her.

In this episode, Jesus put two faith principles into action: he touched her, and he spoke. He issued a command to get up. I don't know, and you don't know, but maybe if he had never said a word, she might never have gotten up off of that bed. Maybe if he had just touched her and had not said a single word, nothing would have happened. But Jesus issued a command: he said, "Get up," and she got up, even though she was dead. She didn't just lie there and say, "I'm dead, I can't do that!" She got up!

In Mark 7:32-35, we read about a time Jesus healed a deaf man: *"And they bring unto him one that was deaf, and had an impediment in his speech; and they beseech him to put his hand upon him. And he took him aside from the multitude, and put his fingers into his ears, and he spit, and touched his tongue; And looking up to heaven, he sighed, and saith unto him, Ephphatha, that is, Be opened. And straightway his ears were opened, and the string of his tongue was loosed, and he spake plain."*

Do you see what Jesus did? He took the man aside from the multitude. He put his fingers in each ear. (HE TOUCHED HIM!) And he commanded those ears to be opened.

He healed those ears by touch, through the power of the Holy Spirit. There are many ways for ears to be healed, but one of the best ones I know is just to stick your fingers in someone's ears and believe the power of God is going to go through those fingers!

At a meeting in Colorado one night, we had a word of knowledge on the healing of ears, and as we touched their ears, 38 out of 39 people were instantly healed. THERE IS POWER IN THE TOUCH!

At a service in Ames, Iowa, a little baby was brought forward whose feet were turned in so badly that the child was horribly crippled. I took one foot in each hand, and while I was holding them, they completely straightened out! I had the thrill of feeling and seeing a miracle in progress. I don't think I even said anything. I just touched the baby, and began to feel the bone structure changing in my hands.

That was not prayer. That was not a command. THAT WAS HEALING THROUGH THE LAYING ON OF HANDS!

We share these personal examples with you because we want to bring your faith up to the point where you will think "Wow, I can do that, too!"

God will often heal more than one person with the same disease in the same meeting, but in different ways. We had a word of knowledge one night for crossed eyes, and three children came forward. One was healed when she came forward. The second one was healed when we put our hands on her eyes. When we removed our hands, the one eye "arced" and settled in the right place.

To the third child we said, "Eyes, be healed in Jesus' name!" She was healed by a command. Three healings, same disease, three different ways!

Sometimes people will be in our services and say, "Charles and Frances can really go out and heal the sick. They just lay hands on them and things happen!"

Charles and Frances Hunter HAVE NO MORE POWER THAN YOU HAVE! But there IS something that may be a little different about us; we USE that power more than most people do. We are two of the most persistent people in the world, because we do not get discouraged like a lot of people do. Before we received the baptism, we laid hands on something like ten thousand people and maybe as many as TEN of them got healed!

We were PERSISTENT even though we didn't realize we needed the baptism with the Holy Spirit.

YOU NEED TO BE PERSISTENT, TOO! If you lay hands on someone, and nothing happens, TRY THE NEXT ONE! Lay hands on him or her. If nothing happens, don't give up! Sometimes Charles and I have ministered to the same person as many as five different ways. We have tried commanding, laying on of hands, casting out devils, but finally the persistence pays off and we see the individual healed!

What if we had said the first time, "I guess this is just not your night," if the person didn't get healed? They might never have been healed! But we kept on being persistent and continued to persevere and to explore areas which are not fully described in the Word of God.

This is what God wants every believer to do: just step out in faith and begin laying hands on the sick, and BELIEVE they are going to recover.

Do you know why I expect the sick to recover when I lay hands on them? Because I believe without a shadow of doubt that Jesus Christ lives his life in and through me. If I did not believe that, there would be no way that people could get healed when I laid hands on them.

Throughout all of his epistles, Paul preached, "Christ IN you, the hope of glory." Paul never portrayed Jesus as being outside of a believer, dragging him along, saying, "Come on, I am going to make you lay hands on the sick. I am going to make you heal them!"

BECAUSE THE WORD OF GOD SAYS IT, WE HAVE TO BELIEVE THAT JESUS CHRIST IS LIVING IN AND THROUGH US! To me, the most exciting thing in the world is to know that the physical body you see when you look at me, is the body that was given to Frances Hunter, but the PERSON WHO LIVES INSIDE is Jesus Christ!

When you fully realize that Jesus is living INSIDE of you, it will totally transform you. Then, one day you will realize that when you put out your hand, it is the hand of Jesus Christ!

Jesus said, *"He that believeth on me, the works that I do shall he do also; and greater works than these shall he do; because I go unto my Father"* (John 14:12). So, who did Jesus leave on this earth to complete his work?

He left us! He commissioned us to lay hands upon the sick, using HIS authority!! Remember, it's all done in the name of Jesus! It is in the name of Jesus that all miracles are done, because Jesus lives in and through us.

That fact does not make us divine, but we do need to know who we are in Christ. When the devil asks you, "Who do you think you are?" You should be able to answer, "I am a child of God. I have the righteousness of God in me. I have Jesus living in my heart. I KNOW who I am! I am not a mere nothing. I am somebody who has Jesus living in me." Each and every born-again, Spirit-filled believer is incredibly important because Jesus is living inside EACH AND EVERY ONE OF US!

Do something for me, will you? Put your hands out in front of you and say, "These are the hands of Jesus, so there is healing power in my hands." Pick your feet up off the floor (not while you're standing) and say, "These are the feet of Jesus! The power of God goes through my entire body. It is not limited to my hands; it is in my feet; it is in my knees; it is in my head; it is all over me!"

Many times because of the size of an audience, Charles and I do not have the opportunity to pray for every individual in a meeting, so we say, "Every person lay hands on yourself!"

THERE IS POWER IN YOUR OWN HANDS TO HEAL YOURSELF! For example, four years ago when we were in Melbourne, Australia, we did this, and said,

"Lay hands on that part of your body which is diseased or afflicted, and God is going to heal you all! That night God had dropped the gift of faith on us, and when we went back to Melbourne four years later, the sponsor of the meeting told us that every person there was healed by laying hands on themselves. Don't ever under-estimate the power of the Holy Spirit which flows through your own hands!

At a recent meeting, I had been laying hands on people who had headaches or migraines, and I said to one woman, "Just lay hands on yourself and say, 'Out in the name of Jesus!'"

When you say, "OUT IN THE NAME OF JESUS," say it with authority! Don't whisper. Let the devil know you have faith! This woman said with great authority, "OUT, IN THE NAME OF JESUS," touched herself on the forehead, and fell over backwards under the power of God!

She had spoken with such authority and belief that she knocked herself right off of her feet, and you never heard an audience laugh like that in your life. When she got up, she said, "My headache disappeared before I ever hit the floor."

THAT IS REAL POWER! That is believing there is power in your hands! Now you go and do the same thing!

By Charles

Have you ever turned a light switch on or off?

If you have, you are smart enough to heal the sick.

Somewhere not too far from where you are there is a generator, a power plant which generates electricity.

This electricity, this power, is brought to your house from the source of the power through a wire, and up to your electric light bulb. The energy which flows from the power plant to the light bulb causes the filament of the bulb to illuminate, and we say the light is on.

Between the power plant and the light bulb is a switch, or a breaker. This switch is designed to break the flow of the energy, the power, from its source to the destination in the light bulb. If you turn the switch "on" the two ends of the wire are connected so the energy will flow through. If it is turned "off," the wire is separated and the energy cannot continue because of the gap between the power source and the light bulb.

In the same way, the Holy Spirit "in you" is the generator or the power plant — the source of the power. Your hands are the on and off switch, and the person needing healing is the light bulb.

Now, it is entirely up to you whether you turn the switch on or off. It is entirely your choice in healing to "lay hands on the sick." The power of God will do the healing, just as the electric current will light the bulb. If you want a dark room light, you can turn the light switch on. If you don't, the room will stay dark. If you have an opportunity to heal someone, it is the same kind of choice. You can lay hands on them and heal them, or let them remain sick!

If you have not yet received your generator, do so right now! Ask Jesus to baptize you with the Holy Spirit, lift your hands up to God, begin to love and praise him, but not in your native language. Start giving sounds of love rapidly so that the Holy Spirit can take those sounds and give you the language which will take any individual and make an extraordinary person out of him! Let your spirit soar as it talks to God for the very first time! (I Cor. 14:2).

Be a "switch" for Jesus, but be sure you are "turned on" for him. Let this be a part of your way of being the light of the world. Jesus said, *"Ye are the light of the world"* (Matt. 5:14).

Laying hands on the sick and healing them is one way Jesus used to be the light of the world — to illuminate the way for the lost to find him. He passed this earth-job on to us, and gave us this healing virtue, this dynamic power in us so we could effectively carry on all of his work while we are on earth.

There is no power in the flesh of our hands, but there is power when God's Holy Spirit flows through our hands!

Our physical bodies are made of dust, or clay. Laying one piece of clay on another piece of clay will not produce any healing results. What we do with our hands may reflect our love and compassion, but only God's power can heal the sick. As human beings, we cannot heal the sick by our own powers.

Our bodies do, however, have the ability to heal themselves. God created us healthy, and he gave us the physical components which will maintain health if we keep the whole realm of our physical body in line with God's laws.

We were in West Texas ministering when a girl thirteen years old came to me for healing. She had fallen at school a year before and a large lump had remained for the whole year. It was still sore, and her mother was very concerned.

I like to pray with my eyes open so I won't miss the exciting miracles. Jesus LOOKED up when he did the exciting miracle of multiplying loaves and fishes into food for thousands.

I had my eyes fixed on the lump and just touched it lightly with my forefinger and said, "In Jesus' name!" The lump disappeared instantly! It was there, and then it was not there!

When you ask Jesus to forgive your sins, he will instantly do it if you mean it when you ask. Before you ask him, your sins are there; and then they are not there, just like that lump!

"Jesus' disciples saw him do many other miracles besides the ones told about in this book, but these are recorded SO THAT YOU WILL BELIEVE THAT HE IS THE MESSIAH, THE SON OF GOD, AND THAT BELIEVING IN HIM YOU WILL HAVE LIFE" (John 20:30,31 TLB).

One night a lady about fifty years old came to me for healing of her nose. She had broken it when she was four or five years old, and it was left crooked like an angle. I softly ran my finger down her nose, and in front of my eyes the bone straightened instantly.

Months later we were having a Mexican dinner with a group of people and I was telling this story. To demonstrate what I did, I ran my finger down the nose of the lady sitting next to me. Her mother, a minister's wife, was sitting across the table from her, and she said, "Look at your nose — it isn't crooked anymore!"

Faith had been brought to her by telling of a miracle, and the power went into her nose by the laying on of a finger and God did a twentieth century miracle. Glory to his mighty name!

Have you noticed that the Bible doesn't say, "Lay hands on the heads of the sick and heal them?" Observe the healings we mentioned and you will see that hands were laid on a nose, on ears, on heads, on hands, on feet, on eyes. Since it is the flow of God's power which heals the sick, we get our hands as close as we can to the part of the body which needs healing. This allows the power to go directly into the sick part. Often the power goes in so strongly that if we touch a foot, the people will go under the power of God.

Another suggestion is to stand as close as possible to the person being healed, because the power actually flows from all parts of your spirit, through all parts of your body, into the person near you. We believe that many are healed in an audience because the faith of believers causes the power of the Holy Spirit in them to become a force field which goes into those around them.

I take any desire of Jesus as seriously as I do a command from God, and therefore I feel just as strongly that we should lay hands on the sick and heal them as I feel about obeying one of the ten commandments.

It is a way Jesus used while on earth to persuade mankind to believe in him as the Messiah, the Savior. The disciples applied the same law, with the same power Jesus used, and we are no different than the disciples, nor in fact, than Jesus was when he was made man for a short time on earth!

What a tremendous privilege!

What an awesome responsibility!

What a trust our Lord Jesus has placed into our hands!

What a great commission he has given us — to actually be his body working here on earth, to do his good will. Jesus died not only to save the lost, but to heal the sick and free the captives from the evils of the devil.

Doing his will is so easy. Just simply lay your hands on the sick and believe that this dynamic power will go forth from the Holy Spirit in you into those who need his touch through you.

If we were translated back to the days when Jesus lived on earth and we had the privilege of being with him, what would we do if he said, "Go catch a fish and take the coin out of its mouth and pay the taxes?" I believe I would outrun Peter to obey him!

Jesus himself set this dynamic way to heal the sick into motion, and he wants us to do it to release hurting humanity and to cause them to believe in him. Jesus said, "... *they shall lay hands on the sick, and they shall recover*" (Mark 16:18). The Living Bible says, "... *and they* (that's you and me) *will be able to place their hands on the sick and heal them.*"

This is spoken directly by Jesus. It is a part of his great commission. THESE ELEVEN WORDS WERE THE LAST RECORDED WORDS HE SPOKE WHILE HE WAS ON EARTH.

Is there a difference in obedience now than then? Jesus has simply said, "Charles, go lay hands on the sick and they will recover for you just like they did for me. Frances, you go lay hands on the sick and I'll heal them through you, too!" He has said the same thing to you, so there should be enough faith in any of us to obey him.

The Word tells us that we Christians are the body of Jesus, so if he did it in a body two thousand years ago, why should we try to change him today?

It is an exciting thing to know that Jesus lives in and through us! It is overwhelming to realize that the same power of the Holy Spirit is always available within us to do miracles.

IF YOU HAVEN'T EXPERIENCED THE THRILL OF SEEING GOD HEAL THROUGH YOUR HANDS, WHY NOT TRY IT!

START RIGHT NOW!

CHAPTER 4

LAYING ON OF HANDS — PLUS!

By Frances

At times we use more than one method to heal the sick. Sometimes we "lay hands" on individuals in accordance with Mark 16:18, then we add to it Mark 11:23-24, which will be "saying" or commanding something to be done; this might be followed by "faith in action"; the "gift of faith" and being slain in the Spirit! You will often discover many different methods are all wrapped up in one healing! So don't stop at one if one way doesn't get them healed!

In the book of Mark, Jesus says, *"And these signs shall follow them that believe ... they shall lay hands on the sick, and they shall recover"* (Mark 16:17,18).

Jesus didn't give us any leeway in that promise. He didn't indicate that there was a probability or possibility of healing; he said THEY WOULD RECOVER, so when we lay hands on you, we expect you to get healed! We believe what Jesus said, and his conditions are simply "those who believe!"

You can even lay hands on yourself, if you're the "sick" one. I do!

If the devil starts to give me a headache, and there's no one around to pray for me, do you know what I do? I lay hands on myself!

The Bible doesn't say, "Those who believe shall lay hands on the sick other than themselves!"

It simply says that those who believe shall lay hands on the sick, and they shall recover. So I lay hands on myself and say, "Headache, out in the name of Jesus!"

Many Christians let the devil rob them of their healings through doubt and unbelief, so don't let doubt sneak in! The minute the devil hears you command an illness to leave, he goes right into action, because he knows Mark 11:23 just as well as you do. He knows you will have whatsoever you say only IF you don't doubt in your heart.

Do you know what kind of personality the devil has? Jesus said, *"He was a murderer from the beginning, and abode not in the truth, because there is no truth in him. When he speaketh a lie, he speaketh of his own: for he is a liar, and the father of it"* (John 8:44). It is the devil's nature to lie to you; it is his nature to try to kill you. Particularly if you have a "fatal" illness, it is the devil's nature to come along with doubt and unbelief after you have been prayed for, because he was a murderer from the beginning.

How does he do it? He tells you, "It didn't work. You're still sick. You don't look like you've been healed at all."

I want to give you a marvelous example to show you how faith works, because I believe that if we can just understand that God's Word is really true — if we will just stand on God's Word (the answer) and not look at the circumstances (the problem), then we will be going in the right direction.

Not too many years ago, a man named Gene Lilly was writing a book on how to die gracefully.

Gene knew he was going to die, because he had been paralyzed for seventeen years and his doctor had told him he was going to die.

He had multiple sclerosis.

He had diabetes.

He had high cholesterol.

He had high triglycerides.

He had scar tissue on the brain.

His body was a mess.

He had listened to a pastor on television one time, and that pastor had pointed a finger right at him and said, "I bet you don't go to church because of the hypocrites."

Gene Lilly said, "That's right! I can't stand hypocrites!"

Gene said that the pastor had an old crooked finger, and he pointed it right at the TV camera, and said, "I'll tell you something about the hypocrites. At least they're doing something. You aren't doing anything!"

As a result of that program, Gene Lilly got saved. Then he thought, "Well, glory to God, I am going to heaven when I die! Even though I have all this pain down here, I am going to suffer gloriously for God, and then I'm going to heaven to be with Jesus." So Gene began writing a book on how to die gracefully when God spoke to him and told him to go to Orlando, Florida.

Gene and his wife lived in Phoenix, Arizona. They didn't know why God had told them to go to Orlando. Gene had quit work to preach the Gospel, and they were so poor they had to sell everything they owned for food and gas money, but they made it to Orlando anyway. And the very first time they went to church there, the pastor preached on "Healing is for you."

After that sermon, Gene began to notice healing scriptures in the Word. One that impressed him was Psalm 107:20, *"He sent his word, and healed them, and delivered them from their destructions."*

Another one was Psalm 118:17, *"I shall not die, but live, and declare the works of the Lord."* He had to check his Bible to make sure that one was in there, because he was still writing the book on how to die gracefully when somebody quoted that scripture to him.

Gene opened his Bible and there it was! His faith began to mount up, and mount up, and mount up, and finally he began to think, "Wow, I could get healed! I really could get healed! According to God's Word, I COULD GET HEALED!" Gene had reached a point where he really believed that healing is for today.

Unfortunately, many people have been told that healing is not for today. According to some, healing was possible back in the days of the disciples, but not today. God does not heal any more. Have you ever heard someone make that statement? IT IS A LIE OF THE DEVIL himself! If Jesus Christ healed yesterday, he will heal today. If he heals today, he will heal tomorrow because he has never changed and never will!

The devil wants you to believe in sickness!

God wants you to believe in healing!

Gene Lilly kept on reading the Bible, and the more he read, the more he began to believe that healing is for today. Then he really got rambunctious, and said, "I believe that healing is not only for today, I believe that healing is for ME!"

Now that's a big step for a man who's writing a book on how to die gracefully!

Next Gene thought, "If I could just meet someone who had ever laid hands on someone and they were healed, they'd know how to pray the prayer of faith for me."

Somebody gave Gene a copy of our book, SINCE JESUS PASSED BY, which tells how God dropped us into the miracle ministry in a Southern Baptist church in El Paso, Texas. Gene said, "Oh, God, if Charles and Frances Hunter would just come to Orlando, Florida, and lay their hands on me, I BELIEVE I WOULD BE HEALED!"

Of course, Gene Lilly didn't need Charles and

Frances Hunter, but he did need a point of contact. He needed something that would release his faith. He had just said to God, "Oh, if I could just meet somebody who had laid hands on the sick and they recovered, I know that if they laid hands on me, then I'd recover too." Now he had just read about some people who had actually had people healed in their ministry.

Gene's faith was rising!

God is good because the very next day, Gene bought a newspaper, and there was a large ad in it which said, "Charles and Frances Hunter will hold a miracle service at the Hilton Inn in Orlando, Florida, right next to Disneyland."

Gene's faith skyrocketed. It literally exploded, because of what he had just said. Here was his opportunity!

The night of the service, Gene's faith was so strong that he said to his wife, "Leave the walker at home! Leave the crutches at home! Leave everything at home, because I'M GOING TO GET HEALED, so you don't need to take any of that stuff along!"

What a way to go to a service!

That night, Gene Lilly's family half-dragged and half-carried him in. We were operating in the gift of word of knowledge (I Cor. 12:8), and called out a healing for a man who was sitting just four or five seats away from him. The man came up and was healed of a deaf ear. Gene was really excited about that, and he kept thinking, "The next one is me! The next one is me!"

Someone else in Gene's row got healed, and then someone over here, and then someone over there, and suddenly he discovered that the miracle service was over and we still had not laid hands on him.

Gene was still just as sick as he ever was!

He was just as paralyzed as he was when he came!

He was just as diabetic as he was when he came!

The multiple sclerosis was just as bad as it was

when he came!

Then I said, "Now, if we did not call out your disease in a word of knowledge, I want you to come forward and you will get healed."

Gene thought, "There it is, there it is!" With almost unbelievable determination, he dragged himself forward, chair by chair, and row by row, until finally he was at the front. Two ushers helped him onto his feet, and held him up!

Gene said, "I have diabetes, I have multiple sclerosis, I have been paralyzed for seventeen years, I have high triglycerides, I have high cholesterol, I have scar tissue on the brain, and I'm dying!"

I said, "Praise Jesus!" And his faith almost went out his feet. Later, Gene told me, "I thought you were the most hardhearted woman I had ever seen in my entire life. Here I tell you I am dying, and you say, 'Praise Jesus!' But then I looked up, and when I saw your eyes, I realized that for the first time in my life I was looking at someone who didn't limit God! When I looked at you, I could see that you BELIEVED that when you laid hands on me, Jesus was going to heal me."

Gene was right. Gene said that every other person had prayed that God would give him grace to stand the suffering in this life until that great day of glory when he would go home to God. Suddenly, he found himself staring into the eyes of a woman who was not limiting God one bit. He said, "I could not believe my ears when I heard that wild prayer you prayed!"

I did not say, "Now God," and go through a long list about the multiple sclerosis, the paralysis, the diabetes, or the other problems. I simply said, "What you need is a Jesus overhaul!" Then I said, "Jesus, overhaul him." And with that, I put my hand on his head, and even with two ushers holding him, the power of God was so strong that he fell flat on his back!

Because his feet were paralyzed, Gene had not been

able to feel shoes for seventeen years. Suddenly his feet began to hurt! His shoes were too small, but he had not known this previously because of the lack of feeling. An excited Gene Lilly knew that God had begun a special work in his body!

After I prayed, Gene struggled to his feet. The ushers helped him up, and if God hadn't spoken to me, I would not have said what I said next, because he went crawling back down the aisle the same way he crawled up.

I said, "He may not look like he is healed, but he is!"

He certainly did not look like he was healed! He was just as crippled, just as paralyzed, and he didn't look one bit better than when he came, but God had spoken to my spirit. I didn't let the devil come in with doubt and unbelief and say, "He does not look to me like he is healed. Sorry about that, folks! Maybe he should come back some other time; he might get healed!" I simply said, "He may not look like he is healed, but he is!" God had given me the gift of faith, and when I said that, Gene Lilly's faith exploded! He believed, and he continued to believe!

Within twelve hours, he was walking like a normal human being, totally healed by the power of God. Even the diabetes was gone. However, I was very emphatic when I told him the same thing we try to tell everyone, "If you are on medication, continue on that medication until the doctor takes you off."

Gene got up the next morning and took his usual shot of insulin, and then he almost went into insulin shock because his body didn't need it any more. He had to drink about a gallon of orange juice, and then he ate candy bars all day to offset the insulin. It was the last insulin he ever took.

Gene's doctor was out of town on Monday, so he called and made an appointment for Tuesday. He told the doctor, "I got healed over the weekend."

The doctor said, "Who healed you?"

"Jesus."

"Jesus who?" the doctor asked.

Hallelujah! Gene Lilly was totally healed by the power of God! What would have happened if he had said to himself that night, "Well, I guess I didn't get it." That is exactly what he would have gotten! He would have gotten, "I guess I didn't get it," because the Bible says that if we believe, we will receive whatever we say.

How did Gene get healed?

By the laying on of hands.

By going under the power of the Holy Spirit.

By the gift of faith in me.

By the gift of faith in Gene.

By a command.

By Gene's putting his faith into action.

You can heal someone by laying on of hands, but since Jesus often used more than one way to heal the sick, sometimes it is wise to use LAYING ON OF HANDS — PLUS!

By Charles

Right after we received the baptism with the Holy Spirit, we began to see an increase in the number of healings in our meetings. The more God did, the more excited we became, and the more we told about his mighty miracles! The more we told about the miracles, the more he did!

One night a man came up on the stage, held up by two people, and leaning heavily on two walking canes. He did not have the strength to lift his feet off the floor; he scooted them along. We asked what affliction he had, and then we prayed (we didn't know at that time that prayer was not really used much as the means of healing). But something else was done!

When we finished praying, instead of saying, "Praise the Lord and go on your way," we said, "PICK UP YOUR CANES AND WALK!" He lifted the canes off the floor and slid his feet forward, and he didn't fall! He tried another step, and he didn't fall! He slid a little more, and still he didn't fall! I took him by the arm and began to walk him a little faster, and a little faster. Then I said, "Bend your knees when you walk." He began to bend his knees, and pretty soon I was running alongside of him across the stage, and he began to say, "Praise the Lord! Hallelujah!" Before we prayed, he spoke so weakly we had to have him repeat his affliction five times before we could understand! But now, it wasn't long before he was yelling so loudly that you could hear him in the back of the room.

What was different about his healing?

We had actually laid our hands on him, BUT we also told him to walk! This was the very first time in our ministry we had told an individual to put his faith into action. And glory to God, he responded and began to exercise his faith. He may not have had a lot, but he had all the faith he needed when he made the first little effort to move his feet and pick up the canes.

Jesus had people put their faith into action!

"Stretch forth thine hand" (Mark 3:5).

"Rise, take up thy bed, and walk" (John 5:8).

"Go, wash in the pool of Siloam" (John 9:7).

We were doing the same thing! Faith needs to be put into action. Healing often takes place at that very instant when people put their faith into action. Laying on of hands PLUS faith in action produces results!

When someone comes up to me with a problem in their elbow, while they are saying, "It was hurt ten years ago, I can't bend it, and it has pain in it," I touch the elbow (laying on of hands) and say, "In the name of Jesus," then quickly say to them, "MOVE YOUR ELBOW, BEND YOUR ELBOW!" When they instantly respond and bend it, even though they are still telling me what is wrong with it, the elbow is totally healed the majority of the time.

Why? Because before they can lose faith, or give me time to lose faith, they have already been healed. Three ways of healing are involved here: Laying on of hands, PLUS a command, PLUS an ACTION OF FAITH!

A national champion cowboy came to one of our services with a real problem for a calf roper. He had injured his shoulder quite seriously and couldn't raise his arm. I reached out like a flash, touched his shoulder and said, "In the name of Jesus, raise your arm!" Without even thinking, he instantly shot his arm straight up, and the expression of surprise on his face was priceless! Prompt faith in action often brings about the desired results because it happens before doubt and unbelief from the devil begin to creep in!

Exciting as this beautiful miracle of God is, the fulfillment of its purpose is even more thrilling. This cowboy is now traveling all over the nation, working in rodeos, telling others how God healed his shoulder —and leading people to Jesus!

Another example of laying on of hands — PLUS: We went to the grand opening of the PTL Club Barn (their great church auditorium), to ride in the parade. We were standing by our float waiting for the parade to start, when we noticed a staff member limping and using a cane.

We asked, "What's wrong with your leg?"

She related an interesting story to us. She had slipped, fallen and broken the bone in her right leg six months before. When the doctor X-rayed it, he noticed it had separated about three-quarters of an inch. He said she would either have to undergo surgery or the leg would be short for the rest of her life.

When the doctor told her that, she said God immediately placed our faces into her mind, and she said, "I'll take my chances, so don't operate."

And here we were right in front of her for the first time since the accident! We found some steps leading up to a float for her to sit on, and held her legs out in front of her. Sure enough, the one leg measured about three-quarters of an inch shorter than the other.

Notice the different healing methods we used. We LAID OUR HANDS ON HER FEET as we held them, and we began to speak to the leg. We COMMANDED the bones to grow together and the leg to grow out in the name of Jesus, and it was a real slowpoke! It took about five minutes for it to grow full length, but it did, and she walked the rest of the day without pain or cane.

Later, she gave a testimony over the PTL television network about God's mighty miracle of putting a bone together out on a hot, windy parade ground!

God gives us many ways to heal the sick, so don't get stuck on using just one way at a time. We have discovered by common sense reasoning in the natural, (Proverbs talks a lot about this) that miracles can happen in the supernatural.

In the case of scoliosis, you need to command a spirit to come out (incurable disease), and then command the bones of the spine to straighten. Even though the spirit comes out, the back doesn't necessarily straighten until the command is given, so if you don't do both, the spine could remain crooked.

A medical doctor in Ohio whose specialty is scoliosis asked us before a service whether or not we had ever seen a scoliosis healing. We related several to him, and invited him to participate in the healing service to help us learn and understand what God was doing.

We asked everyone in the audience of 4,000 to 5,000 people to check their arms to see if they were uneven, indicating some kind of back, neck, hip or shoulder problem. We estimated that over 700 indicated by remaining standing that they had short arms. We asked the ushers to select ten people with what we call "goodies" which are sufficiently different in length to be easily seen from the stage. The doctor was on the stage with us, and one of those who came up had scoliosis which she said was about a thirty-degree curvature. The left arm of the girl was about three or four inches shorter than the right.

The doctor stood with us as we commanded the spirit of scoliosis to come out in the name of Jesus AND commanded the arm to grow. The arm grew out even with the other, so we asked the doctor to check her to see what happened to the back. He could only do a limited examination without an X-ray and proper examining equipment. He had her bend forward as he ran his hand down her spine. He said it seemed to him that there was still about a ten-degree curvature.

We had her remain in the bent-over position as we did the next step in the healing. The doctor held the microphone so he could talk to the audience as we commanded the spine to straighten, in the name of Jesus! A hush came over the audience, then exciting enthusiasm filled the entire auditorium as this medical specialist said, "It's moving! It's moving! It's moving!" A long silence followed as he continued running his hand up and down her spine. Finally he said, "It appears to me to be straight!" Hallelujah!

Two days later a call came into our office from the girl's personal physician. He said, "Send me every tape and book you have about this. I have never seen such a thing in my life! The spine is perfectly straight!"

These same exciting miracles are in your future, too, WHEN YOU LAY HANDS ON PEOPLE — PLUS!

CHAPTER 5

LET THE SICK LAY HANDS ON YOU!

By Frances

"Everyone was trying to touch him, for when they did healing power went out from him and they were cured" (Luke 6:19 TLB).

And whithersoever he entered, into villages, or cities, or country, they laid the sick in the streets, and besought him that they might touch if it were but the border of his garment: and as many as touched him were made whole" (Mark 6:56).

Jesus didn't need to touch them; they touched him and were healed because the power of the Holy Spirit, which is like a wind or energy, flowed out of him into them!

"But ye shall receive power, after that the Holy Ghost is come upon you" (Acts 1:8).

Was it Jesus who healed the people? Yes and no! Jesus was God's earthly container, but it was the power of God's Holy Spirit that did the healing.

We, too, can be those earthly containers for the power of God to flow through, because this is a scriptural method of healing which is the opposite of laying hands on the sick.

Let the sick lay hands on you! There are not very many examples of this type of healing in the Bible, and

I haven't heard of too many present-day examples of it, but there are times when it does happen.

"And a certain woman, which had an issue of blood twelve years, and had suffered many things of many physicians, and had spent all that she had, and was nothing bettered, but rather grew worse, when she had heard of Jesus, came in the press behind, and touched his garment. For she said, if I may touch but his clothes, I shall be whole. And straightway the fountain of her blood was dried up; and she felt in her body that she was healed of that plague. And Jesus, immediately knowing in himself that virtue had gone out of him, turned him about in the press, and said, 'Who touched my clothes?' And his disciples said unto him, Thou seest the multitude thronging thee, and sayest thou, Who touched me? And he looked round about to see her that had done this thing. But the woman fearing and trembling, knowing what was done in her, came and fell down before him, and told him all the truth. And he said unto her, Daughter, thy faith hath made thee whole; go in peace, and be whole of thy plague" (Mark 5:25-34). This woman knew that she was healed.

You need to know HOW TO HEAL, but you also need to know what to say to people who have a negative attitude. For example, fairly often someone will come up to us and say "Will you pray for my Aunt Jane?"

I will say, "Is Aunt Jane here? I would love to pray for her."

"No, she was too sick to come."

Too sick to come! Let me tell you this. If Aunt Jane called a doctor, and the doctor said, "I am calling an ambulance, and I am taking you to the hospital," Aunt Jane would be in the hospital as soon as the ambulance could get her there! Generally, it is a weak excuse to say, "Aunt Jane is too sick to come." If you are too sick to come, that is when you need to have hands laid on you!

The woman who touched the hem of Jesus' garment could have looked for excuses. She could have said, "I have been to every doctor in the world and nothing has done me any good, so what is the sense of trying to get up to this man Jesus? I might as well die and get it over with!" Do you think there are people like that today? There certainly are!

Not too long ago, the Spirit of God told me that there was a man in our service who had very severe emphysema, and that he was going to die if God's healing touch was not on him. Although I announced this, the man did not come forward for laying on of hands. As Charles and I were leaving the service, I said to him, "May I pray for you?" He said, "No, I am doing my own thing with God. If God wants to do it, he will do it!"

Well, do you lay hands on someone like that? No, because it would not do any good if you did. That is the same kind of individual who would say, "I am not going to pray the sinner's prayer, because if God wants to save me, let him save me!" He would never get saved, would he?

Here is another one of my pet peeves. "I have been prayed for by the best. I have been prayed for by Kenneth Hagin, Kenneth Copeland, Kathryn Kuhlman, Oral Roberts, Jim Bakker, Pat Robertson, Rex Humbard ..." and on and on. Then they'll say, "Will you pray for me?"

What good would it do if I prayed? None, because there are some people who just like to come forward so they can go around naming all the great evangelists who have unsuccessfully laid hands on them. But they never believe anything is going to happen!

The woman who touched the hem of Jesus' garment could have said the same thing. "All these great doctors tried to heal me, and it didn't do any good."

She could have looked at that crowd and said, "What a mess, I am not going to try. Why, there is no way I can get through to Jesus. It must not be God's will for me to be healed!"

There are all kinds of excuses people can make. But she didn't make excuses! I see her as a woman of great persistence. She probably had come a long way to get there, and could have said, "I might as well go home. I did all that traveling for nothing. I can't even get close to him."

But she didn't. I imagine she stood there like a race horse. She probably started pawing the ground with her feet, saying, "Let me out of here, let me into that crowd. I am going to get there. I don't care what I have to do. I don't care if I have to crawl on my knees to get there. Whatever it takes, I am going to get to Jesus, and I am going to touch the hem of his garment, because I know that when I do I am going to be healed by the power of God!"

That woman could have used every excuse in the world, but she didn't!

She could have let circumstances discourage her, but she didn't!

She could have reached out and thought, "I will get in trouble if I touch that man."

She could have let fear take over, but she did not! She was determined that there was one thing she had to do, and that was all! She was determined to touch the hem of that garment, because she KNEW that when she did, she was going to be made whole! And because she was persistent, SHE WAS HEALED!

Her FAITH in that case was TOUCHING IN RE-VERSE. She didn't even ask if Jesus would touch her. She just said, "If I can just touch HIM, I will be made whole."

And she was!

This is a beautiful Bible story, but who has that much power in his clothing today? Who is walking around today with so much resurrection power that someone can come up and touch him or a piece of his clothing and get healed?

What is the answer to that question? EACH AND EVERY SPIRIT-FILLED BELIEVER HAS THE SAME RESURRECTION POWER IN HIM!

Here is the story of the hem of another garment.

I have been a fanatic from the day I was saved. I say that joyfully, because when Jesus Christ came into my heart, I KNEW that he came in. I KNEW I was a new creature. I KNEW that old things had passed away! I KNEW that all things had become new! I KNEW I was saved! I KNEW that Jesus was living in my heart!

It was the wildest, most exciting thing in the world to KNOW that Jesus was in me. I felt like going around saying, "Look, look, can you see him? He is living inside of me!"

Years ago, even before I received the baptism with the Holy Spirit, exciting things had been happening because I was totally committed to God. One of the greatest, most important things in the whole world is that total complete sellout to God when you don't care what anyone thinks about you, you don't care what happens, as long as you can just serve God and do what God wants you to do.

I had come back from a trip, and in my home church, which did not believe in the baptism with the Holy Spirit, I was sharing some of the exciting things that had happened, how God had used me, and how hundreds and hundreds of people had accepted Jesus as their Savior and Lord.

At the end of the service, a little note was handed to me which said, "There is a woman in our congregation who is very ill, and she asked if you would stop by her house on your way home." I agreed, and when I entered the house, I saw the woman lying on just a plain mattress on the floor.

I didn't know very much about healing at that time.

I KNEW that God healed, but I wasn't sure exactly how he did it. I didn't have any power, but blind simple faith will do a lot!

When I came through the door, she said, "Would you do just one thing for me?"

I said, "Certainly, I will do whatever you want."

She said, "Would you stand right over here?" Her voice was so weak, and she began to inch across the mattress until she got right to the very edge. Then she said, "Would you come real close to me?"

I said, "Sure." She had not asked me to pray.

She said, "Would you get a little closer?"

I kept getting a little closer, but I didn't understand what she wanted. Suddenly, she looked up at me with the most beautiful faith that I have ever seen in the eyes of any grown person. She said, "If I could just touch the hem of your garment, I KNOW that I would be made whole."

I looked down at my dress and thought, "It sure does not look very special to me!" It did not look the least bit anointed to me! But this woman felt exactly the same way the woman in the Bible did.

She reached out and touched the hem of the skirt that I was wearing, and when she did she was instantly made whole by the power of God!

That was some fourteen years ago. I saw her the last time I was back in Florida, and she has had no recurrence of that horrible cancer that was causing her to hemorrhage to death. She is an extremely healthy, active woman today.

God had put faith into that woman. That faith said, "Just touch the hem of Frances' garment." She didn't even ask to touch me. She could have touched my leg more easily than she touched my dress, but somehow her faith was in touching the hem of my dress.

There is absolutely nothing special about anything I ever wear! Absolutely nothing! But when you are committed to God, you are anointed! Your skin is anointed, your body is anointed, your hands and your feet are anointed! You have been anointed to heal the sick, therefore any piece of clothing that touches you is equally anointed!

"And God did unusual and extraordinary miracles by the hands of Paul, so that handkerchiefs or towels or aprons which had touched his skin were carried away and put upon the sick, and their diseases left them, and the evil spirits came out of them" (Acts 19:11, 12 Amp.).

Most people don't realize it, but that happens to be just one very unique and scriptural way to heal the sick.

CHAPTER 6
TALK TO A MOUNTAIN!!!

By Frances

In Mark 11:23 Jesus says, *"For verily I say unto you, That whosoever shall say unto this mountain, Be thou removed, and be thou cast into the sea; and shall not doubt in his heart, but shall believe that those things which he saith shall come to pass; he shall have whatsoever he saith."*

Jesus is saying this to YOU! Whosoever is you! Whosoever is ME! Whosoever is EVERYONE! God is no respecter of persons. He simply says, "whosoever."

This particular verse is very important because it has a lot to do with ONE way of healing. It says, "Whosoever shall SAY."

It does not say, "Whosoever shall pray!"

It says, "Whosoever shall SAY!"

And there is a BIG difference between SAYING and PRAYING!

When you SAY unto this mountain, "Be thou cast into the sea," you are COMMANDING that mountain to do something, because you know who you are in Christ! You have the power of God IN you, and you are operating the way the Bible tells you to operate. Speak with authority at all times if you want to see miracles happen. This doesn't mean you have to yell and scream (we tried that, too!) but it does mean to speak with authority so that the devil knows that you know you have power!

When you PRAY, you are asking God to do something.

When you SAY, YOU are commanding something to be done!

Are you aware of the fact that the disciples never prayed for the sick after they received the baptism with the Holy Spirit? Jerry Horner, professor of theology at Oral Roberts University, is one of the greatest Bible scholars we know, and he said that to his knowledge there is NO RECORDED PLACE IN THE BIBLE WHERE THE DISCIPLES EVER PRAYED FOR THE SICK AFTER THE DAY OF PENTECOST! Jesus didn't pray for the sick! The disciples didn't pray for the sick, so why should we?

After Paul shook off the viper and felt no evil effects, he was ministering healing to Publius, the father of the head man of the island. *"... and Paul went to see him, and AFTER PRAYING and laying his hands on him HE HEALED HIM"* (Acts 28:8 Amp.). It is scriptural to pray before we minister healing. Please don't get legalistic about this, however, and feel that if you do pray you are not scriptural.

Jesus said that all authority in heaven and earth had been given to him (Matt. 28:18), and then he turned around and gave us his authority to cast out devils and lay hands on the sick and heal them.

Several years ago we had been ministering at the Willamette Christian Center in Eugene, Oregon, when God started a beautiful miracle of "saying!" Because our services are sometimes a little different than the ordinary church service, a few people in a congregation might tend to get "up tight" because we praise God in the dance, or are extremely enthusiastic about the things God does! As a result, every year after we leave, Pastor Murray McLees always "soothes the ruffled feathers" of anyone in his congregation who might not understand the charismatic movement.

This particular year he made an unusual statement to his congregation. He said something like this: "You might not always agree with everything Charles and Frances Hunter do, but I'll tell you one thing. If I ever get sick, I wouldn't want anyone but Charles and Frances to pray for me because their faith is so simple, they just believe if they lay hands on you, you will be healed! And you will be!"

Little did he realize he was prophesying about his very own life! Shortly after this, the devil laid a "killer" brain tumor on him which was one of the fastest-growing types of cancer known. Before long, he was blind in one eye, and deaf in one ear, and had excruciating pain in his head.

God placed into remembrance in the mind of a woman in his congregation what Murray had said about who he wanted to pray for him if he ever got sick, so she miraculously got our unlisted telephone number and called us to let us know what Pastor McLees had shared with his congregation that very morning. THE DOCTORS HAD ONLY GIVEN HIM A MONTH OR TWO TO LIVE! His congregation was devastated by the news!

He resigned from all his community affairs, and they credited him with perfect attendance as was their custom for individuals with terminal illnesses. Pastor McLees said he had always had faith to pray for himself and other people, but this time his faith went right out the window, and I'm sure we've all experienced the same thing at one time or another!

We immediately called him, and the Spirit of God emphatically told us we were not to go to him, but to bring him to one of our miracle services. We told him what the Spirit had said and told him we would pay his way and his wife's way to any miracle service he would choose in the United States. I'll never forget his reply. He said, "That blends with my spirit!" They chose San Diego, California, as THEIR miracle service because it was only about ten days away!

They did not arrive until the last service, and then they were late. When we saw them come in, we left the stage and ran over and hugged them. Our hearts were breaking because of what the devil had done to our beloved brother in Christ. We did not pray at that moment simply because we were not led to do anything except show him the love of God.

We returned to the stage with Pastor Jerry Barnard for additional worship, and as Pastor Barnard was ministering in the word of knowledge the Lord spoke to me and said, "Pray for him RIGHT NOW!" I turned to ask Charles to go get Murray, but he had already gone, and when I turned back, Pastor Barnard had turned to me to tell Charles to bring Murray to the stage. The Spirit of God had spoken to ALL of us at the SAME TIME!

Charles brought Pastor McLees to the center of the ballroom at El Cortez Hotel where the meeting was being held, and I laid hands on him and spoke to that mountain! And I spoke it with all the authority I know belongs to me as a believer, because I was mad at the devil for what he was trying to do to one of God's children! I said, "Devil, I bind you in the name of Jesus and by the power of God, and I cut ALL your power off. Now you evil, foul spirit of cancer you come out of Murray RIGHT NOW IN THE NAME OF JESUS!"

Pastor McLees fell under the power of God, and so did his wife. It was an emotional moment for all of us! The TV cameras which had been turned on him, came back on me when he fell under the power, and I shouted at the top of my lungs, "Turn the camera back on him, because I want the world to see what a man looks like when he's being healed of terminal cancer!"

A gasp went through the audience as the Spirit moved on everyone! Some thought I was calling into being something that did not exist, just as though it did! Some thought I had received the gift of faith, but it didn't happen to be either, although you can see we had spoken to a mountain to move! What really happened was a vision, because I saw the fingers of God descend into Pastor McLees' brain, and these divine fingers squeezed the tumor right out of his brain! I could see it being squeezed out as plainly as I can see the pages of this book. It almost looked like the fingers were pushing it out of every crack and crevice in his brain!

He got up off the floor with no visible evidence of anything having happened, except he said, "My head doesn't hurt any more!" They returned to their seats and sat down. Before long he looked at his wife and said, "I can see the color in Frances' dress!" And by the next morning, after God had moved on his body the whole night long, his sight had returned to normal as well as his hearing!

Instead of going home to die, three months later he went to Sri Lanka. The first person he prayed for did not have an eyeball, and when he laid hands on him, an eyeball formed in his eye!

When Murray returned to the doctor, the doctor made an X-ray to see what was going on, and his report was, "It looks to me like THAT TUMOR HAS BEEN SQUEEZED RIGHT OUT OF YOUR BRAIN! THE SAC IT WAS IN IS COMPLETELY EMPTY!" Glory to God! The doctor verified exactly what God had shown me in a vision!

I hate the devil with every ounce of strength I have, and when I spoke to the mountain, there was no doubt I meant business. Notice that I did not pray, but I really did SAY it!

This same principle also works in reverse, so we need to watch what we say with our mouth! Christians have brought the most horrible things on themselves simply by the words they have said, because Jesus didn't put any limitations on this promise. He didn't say, "He shall have whatsoever he saith if it's good for him," he said, "He shall have WHATSOEVER he saith."

Let me give you a very good example. When I lived in Florida, a wave of flu came through every October, and EVERY October I had enough faith to move a mountain, even though I wasn't saved at the time. Do you know what the mountain was? It was my health. I had enough faith to change my normally healthy self into a flu victim. I did it with my own big mouth, and didn't even realize what I was doing.

On the first of October, this was my typical comment: "Well, here it is October again, and every October I get the flu. It doesn't make any difference if it is the Asian flu, the Hong Kong flu, swine flu, horse flu; it doesn't make any difference what it is, I GET IT!!"

I was snared by the words of my own mouth! I had absolutely no doubt in my mind whatsoever that I was going to get the flu, regardless of the kind of flu it was.

Then I would go on to an even greater act of faith, and SAY with authority: "It doesn't make any difference what I do. I can go to the doctor fifty times; he can give me penicillin; he can give me B-12; it won't do a bit of good, because I am going to be flat on my back for three solid weeks regardless of what I do!"

Guess where I spent October every year! I spent it in bed, not because other people were catching the flu, but because of my own mouth. I didn't have to come down with the flu, but I was operating by the principles of Mark 11:23. I SAID it and I BELIEVED it! There was not one bit of doubt in my heart whatsoever. I knew I was going to catch the flu. AND I DID!

Glory to God! I AM NEVER GOING TO HAVE THE FLU AGAIN!

I got saved, learned what the Word of God says, and

now I don't need to have the flu, because if the devil tries to bring it around my house, I say, "Take it somewhere else, devil, I don't want it here. I am not signing for that package. Don't leave it an my house, because I don't want any of that." AND I SAY IT WITH AUTHORITY!

Do you see what I am saying with my mouth? You can say the same thing. Mark 11:23 is just as true for you as it is for me. I am "whosoever" and you are "whosoever." When Jesus said "whosoever," he meant that each and every servant of God who believes that verse can say, "Be thou removed and be thou cast into the sea," and if he doesn't doubt in his heart, he will have whatever he says.

Why do so many people find it so easy to believe the devil instead of God? Why is it that people believe bad things are going to happen instead of good ones? The devil comes around with tiny little symptoms, and it's such a temptation to say, "Oh, I'm coming down with something."

Stop right there! Now is the time for the greater one who is in you to rise up and say, "Oh, no you don't, devil! I am not looking at the circumstances, and I am certainly not looking at the symptoms. I am looking at what the Word of God says, and the Word says that if I want a mountain moved, I can have that mountain moved — and the mountain I'm moving now is sickness. Sickness — did you hear me?"

We hope you noticed what Mark 11:23 says to talk "to."

Does it tell us to talk to God?

Does it say, "Pray to God and ask him to get the mountain out of the way?"

No, it says, "Whosoever shall say UNTO THIS MOUNTAIN."

You need to talk to the disease itself. If it's flu, you need to say, "Flu, get out! I am not the least bit interested in your cluttering up my body. I have no time for you. I have too many things to do, so go away in Jesus' name!" If it's cancer, speak to the cancer! If it's the back, speak to the back.

TALK TO THE DISEASE! Speak with authority and then believe! Throw out doubt and don't let unbelief creep in through wavering and listening to the devil, because the next condition is, "and shall not doubt in his heart, but shall BELIEVE that those things which he saith shall come to pass ..."

Doubt and unbelief ALWAYS come from the devil! Any time you hear a voice that speaks doubt and unbelief, don't listen, because it's the DEVIL himself! God never speaks doubt!

Commanding a disease to go, or a body to straighten up is one of the easiest ways to heal the sick. During the past few years, there has been confusion and misunderstanding at times between "saying" and "confessing." These are two different areas of healing. One is doing — the other is receiving. Let's see if we can help clarify the difference between the two:

SAYING is a command to be healed!

CONFESSING is believing for a future act or manifestation of the healing.

There is a vast difference between the two. SAYING is giving authority to words, and CONFESSING is receiving the promise; both confessing and saying are calling into being something that does not exist at the present time.

Both are great, but don't get them confused. Problems have arisen because of this. Isaiah 53:5, *"But he was wounded for our transgressions, he was bruised for our iniquities: the chastisement of our peace was upon him; and with his stripes we are healed,"* has become a well-known scripture to all.

Christians need to exercise faith when they use this healing method, but they also need to exercise discretion. Let me give you an example: One time a young man was having an epileptic seizure. He was foaming at the mouth, his body was doing all sorts of contortions on the floor, and as we ran over to lay hands on him, he became almost violent, and a friend of his said, "Don't lay hands on him, because he's healed!"

There happened to be someone there who was not a Christian, and this guy looked at us and said, "Do you believe that?" It totally turned this man off, because he didn't understand. He just looked at what he saw, and he thought, "Wow! All that foam is coming out of his mouth, someone is getting a pencil to stick in his mouth so he won't swallow his tongue, his body is all contorted, and they're saying this guy is healed?"

After the seizure was over, the man said, "Why did you pray for me? I'm healed by his stripes!" Remember, Jesus healed the sick so people would believe!

The man who was having the seizure meant well, and so did his friend, but he did not use wisdom in what he said, since he was talking to someone who wasn't saved. Because the man was an unbeliever, his faith level was nonexistent. "Claiming" healing has turned off a lot of people because they say, "If you say you are healed even though you are still foaming at the mouth and having contortions on the floor, then either you've lost your marbles, or you don't serve a very good God. Thanks just the same, but I don't want your religion — I think I'll try another one."

We need to exercise discretion. When you say you are healed by the stripes of Jesus, say it to someone whose faith and understanding is on the same or a higher level than yours, and your own faith will build! Never say to an unbeliever that you are healed when the manifestation is not there. It is more correct to say, "I BELIEVE I receive my healing." The best person to say it to is yourself! Keep saying it to yourself until your faith level is built up to the point where you can honestly believe it and receive it, and once you've received it, you can go out and say, "By his stripes I was healed." I personally think it's even better to confess it to God!

How do we get to the point where we believe what we confess? I read a book one time that said, "When you finish reading this book, I want everybody to raise your hands and say every morning, 'God, I love you.' Tomorrow when you get up say, 'God, I love you.' Get up the next morning and say, 'God, I love you.'"

The first time I said that, I thought, "God, I don't know if I do or not. I know that you love me. I know that you let Jesus die so that I might have eternal life. I accept your love for me, but I don't know if I really love you or not. God I love you."

I still didn't know if I believed that or not, but I thought I'd try it again the next morning. I got up and said, "God, I love you." I paused and added, "Hmm, I don't know if I love you or not!" I still didn't feel like I loved him. Both Charles and I have always been honest with God, because God knows what we're thinking anyway. So I kept on for thirty days saying, "God, I love you. I don't know if I really do or not, but God, I love you."

Then one morning, I got up and said, "God, I love you." And then I said, "Oh, God, I really do! I REALLY DO LOVE YOU! Not only do I accept your love for me, but I LOVE YOU!"

How did I get to the point where I really loved God? I kept on making a confession of my love for God. I kept on saying, "God I love you," until it became a reality in my life; until it got into my spirit.

Now can you understand the principle behind saying, "With his stripes we are healed"? We need to be honest with God, because we can't fool him by saying, "With his stripes I am healed. I am putting you on the spot, God, because I said it and now you have to heal me." No, he doesn't! He doesn't have to do a thing unless you really believe without a shadow of a doubt that you were healed. But do you know what? If you keep on saying it, one day, just as I became aware of the fact that I really did love God, you will suddenly realize that YOU HAVE BEEN HEALED! In the meantime, if you are on medication, stay on it so you will live until you are healed!

For several years, I had a great big dark spot on my face, and every time we went on television, I had to cover it up with heavy makeup. Even so, I could still see that dark spot through the makeup. One day I thought, "This really isn't God's best! The Word of God says that I am healed." So I put my finger on the dark spot and said, "Jesus, touch it."

The next day, I looked at the dark spot and it hadn't faded a bit! So I said, "Thank you, Jesus. By your stripes I am healed."

The next day when I put on my makeup, I said, "Thank you, Jesus, by your stripes I am healed."

Then one day, I forgot to say it! Do you know why? BECAUSE IT WASN'T THERE ANY MORE!

If this way works for you, great! Keep on doing it! But if it doesn't work for you, don't feel bad about trying another one of God's provisions.

You may be thinking, "Doesn't that indicate a lack of faith?" No, it does not indicate a lack of faith; it indicates a lot of intelligence! Many, many people are healed simply because they quote the Word of God until they believe, but that's not the only way God has of healing us!

Here's an interesting example. We were ministering in the state of Washington one time, and a lady came to the service in a wheel chair.

She said, "My church teaches that once you have had hands laid on you, you should never go back and be prayed for again, because that indicates a lack of faith." For years, she told us, she had been saying, "By his stripes I am healed."

"Are you walking?" I asked her.

"No!"

"Then you are not healed. The provision is there for your healing, but THERE IS A GREAT DIFFERNCE BETWEEN THE PROVISION AND THE MANIFESTATION.

The provision was there for me to be saved 64 years ago when I was born, but do you know what? It took me 49 years to get around to accepting the provision that was made for my salvation.

The provision for my salvation was available all that time, but I was not saved until I BELIEVED, and accepted my salvation. Even though the provision was valid, my salvation was not, because I hadn't accepted that provision.

What if I had gone to church just one time, and come home and said, "Well, I didn't get saved. So I guess it is not God's will for me to be saved. I went to church once and I did not get saved."

Actually I went to church three times a week for nine months before I got saved, because it was so hard to get me to confess that I was a sinner. But, praise the Lord for my persistence, because I kept on going until I believed in my heart, until it got into my spirit, and in the twinkling of an eye I was saved.

This woman said, "They tell me if I get prayed for once more, it will be showing a lack of faith. They say if you get prayed for once then you are already healed unless you have a lack of faith or sin in your life."

I said, "Do you know what I would do if I were you? Honey, I'd get in every prayer line I could find until I walked!"

"What about that scripture, 'By whose stripes ye were healed?'" she asked.

"That is one way," I told her, "but let's try another way!"

That evening, we asked for those who wanted hands laid on them to come forward, and this woman came. I laid hands on her in Jesus' name, and she sat there like a bump on a log. Some people from her church got hold of her the next day and said, "See, you didn't get healed. You'll never get healed now, because you showed a lack of faith when you went forward last night."

The next day, this woman didn't come. She cried all day long. We were going to be there one more day, and she came to the morning service. She got there early, hoping to talk to us before the service started. She said, "I don't know what to do. They all jumped on me yesterday, and told me that I had sin in my life, because I went forward for prayer again. They keep telling me that since I've been prayed for I already am healed. But I just think I am not healed."

I asked her, "Have you been walking this morning?"

"No," she answered.

"Then," I said, "the provision is still there, but you are still not healed. You come forward at the end of the service this morning. You never know when YOUR day is going to be."

Through tears, she asked, "Do you really think it is all right if I come forward again?"

"Sure," I said, "if I were you I would not quit. I would be the most persistent person God ever had. I believe God would heal me just to get rid of me, because I would keep on knocking at his door until it opened."

At the end of the service, she came forward. I laid hands on her and quoted that wonderful scripture in Acts 3:6: *"Silver and gold have I none; but such as I have give I thee: In the name of Jesus Christ of Nazareth rise up and walk."*

DO YOU KNOW WHAT SHE DID? Even though she had been shot in the back and her spinal cord was severed, she stood up and walked right out of that wheel chair! HALLELUJAH!

You see, God had provided for her healing 2,000 years ago, and she had been quoting that scripture for years. But if we had said to her, "That's great! That's all you need, keep on quoting that," she might still be in the wheel chair. We took pictures of her as she put her healthy husband in the wheel chair and pushed him out of the church. Hallelujah!

Thank God, there is more than one way to heal the sick! If you are quoting scripture for your healings, and it works, keep right on doing it! And if you teach other people to get healed that way, and it works, keep right on teaching it. But if one particular method hasn't worked for you, try another one. God doesn't limit himself to just one way of healing people, so why should you?

God can heal you any way he wants!

We have seen people come forward and say, "When you laid hands on me, I was just standing there, and this tremendous cloud came all over me, and I felt like a piece of jelly. All of a sudden, I could feel every corpuscle in my body moving, and before I knew it I was totally healed!" I suppose that's one way people get healed, but it's not the only way. Everyone does not have to turn into jelly and have a cloud come over them!

We have seen people go under the power of God and be instantly healed while they're lying on the floor.

We have seen people who didn't go under the power of God who were healed standing up.

We have seen people who went under the power of God and didn't get healed.

We've seen people who stayed on their feet and didn't get healed.

God can do whatever he wants, whenever he wants! He can even heal you on the way home from a meeting. You don't have to be in church to be healed, because God can heal you any place he wants.

God can not only heal you any place he wants, he

can heal you regardless of your problem. God can heal a wart, or he can heal a broken toe just as easily as he can heal cancer. In some of our meetings, we have seen cancers actually fall right off, but God doesn't heal them all that way.

We have also seen people vomit them up. But in the long run it's not important whether a cancer fell out, or was vomited out, or simply disappeared. The important thing is that there's no more cancer in that person's body!

Whether you SAY it or CONFESS it, or however you get healed or heal others, remember the one important thing, *"And now, through Christ, all the kindness of God has been poured out upon us undeserving sinners; and now he is sending us out around the world to TELL ALL PEOPLE EVERYWHERE THE GREAT THINGS GOD HAS DONE FOR THEM, SO THAT THEY, TOO, WILL BELIEVE AND OBEY HIM"* (Rom. 1:5 TLB).

CHAPTER 7

WHAT YOU SEE IS WHAT YOU GET!

By Frances

Praise God that the eyes of our understanding are open for new spirit revelations because God is always right there wanting us to have a greater understanding of his Word and his workings.

One of the most outstanding teachings that has been received by the body of Christ has been from Mark 11:23 and 24, *"For verily, I say unto you, That whosoever shall say unto this mountain, Be thou removed, and be thou cast into the sea; and shall not doubt in his heart, but shall believe that those things which he saith shall come to pass; he shall have whatsoever he saith. Therefore I say unto you, What things soever ye desire, when ye pray, believe that ye receive them, and ye shall have them."*

I believe there is a dimension to this scripture which will take us into another realm of healing. The eyes of our understanding are being enlightened, and I believe that as we go into the final stages before Jesus Christ comes back again, people are going to be looking into the spirit world as they have never looked into that vast, exciting world before!

I believe that God is going to open our spirit eyes! We are going to see a lot more angelic activities! Many people who never dreamed that an angel would ever come down in the twentieth century are going to be surprised to see angels accompanying them wherever they go.

We will see the supernatural power of God greatly accelerate where healing is concerned!

I believe the supernatural power of God will be operating through great hosts of ordinary people. For many years, we had only a few "stars" who went out and laid hands on the sick. God is no respecter of persons, so there are no "stars" in the kingdom of heaven, but I believe that God is raising up armies of people all over the world to go out and lay hands upon the sick!

The more we learn about the different ways to heal the sick, the more qualified we will be to go out. We want to remind you that if one thing does not work, try something else until you have victory in that area.

I want to share something with you that I have not totally developed yet, but I believe you can see from some of the things which have happened as a result of this revelation that it opens up a whole new world for healing. I believe you will find this a real bell-ringer in your own life!

Look at the second chapter of II Kings: *"And it came to pass, when the Lord would take up Elijah into heaven by a whirlwind, that Elijah went with Elisha from Gilgal. And Elijah said unto Elisha, Tarry here, I pray thee; for the Lord hath sent me to Beth-el. And Elisha said unto him, As the Lord liveth, and as thy soul liveth, I will not leave thee."* I want you to remember that phrase, because it is very important! *"So they went down to Beth-el. And the sons of the prophets that were at Beth-el came forth to Elisha, and said unto him, Knowest thou that the Lord will take away thy master from thy head to day? And he said, Yea, I know it; hold ye your peace."*

Watch the words that Elijah said, then note the answer by Elisha, and watch for repetition.

"And Elijah said unto him, Elisha, tarry here, I

pray thee; for the Lord hath sent me to Jericho. And he said, As the Lord liveth, and as thy soul liveth, I will not leave thee. So they came to Jericho." Did you notice the repetition again?

"And the sons of the prophets that were at Jericho came to Elisha, and said unto him, Knowest thou that the Lord will take away thy master from thy head today? And he answered, Yea, I know it; hold ye your peace. And Elijah said unto him, Tarry, I pray thee, here; for the Lord hath sent me to Jordan. And he said, As the Lord liveth, and as thy soul liveth, I will not leave thee. And they two went on."

I want to stop just one little moment there, because this is so vital in your Christian experience. Elijah kept saying to Elisha, "Get lost!" Notice he kept saying, "Tarry here, I am going over to so and so, you just stay here, Buddy!" Elisha knew that Elijah had something that he wanted, and he was not about to miss out on the blessing of God. And he kept saying, "Oh, no, you don't, Brother. As long as you live, I'm not going to leave you. As the Lord lives and as you live, I am not going to leave you. Here I come." And so Elisha went along with him.

Elisha was one of the most persistent men in the Bible, and I want you to be the most persistent follower of Jesus Christ that the world has ever known; because God is looking for people who have persistence! God will give you power, but God is looking for people with persistence.

Persistence pays off in every area of your life. I don't care what area you are operating in, persistence will pay off.

I want to show you a really good example of that. I was born with persistence! I lived with persistence. If you could see me in person, you might find it difficult to believe, but I weighed only two pounds when I was born. My first bed was a shoe box, believe it or not, because that is how small I was. No one believed that my parents would ever raise me. Praise God! I sure proved them wrong!

There was a little thread of persistence in there that was hanging on, and hanging on, and it said, "I want to live, I want to live!" Persistence is so vital! This has been with me my whole life long, and I praise God for the characteristic of persistence. Persistence brings success! I have never known anyone who was a success who was not persistent.

Many times people get sidetracked because they lay hands on the sick one time, and when that one person doesn't get healed, they say, "Well, God didn't call me into a healing ministry."

The first person I ever prayed for died! But that didn't keep me down. I thought, "Well, surely I will get a better track record!" You cannot do any worse than that, can you? That should not discourage you. You should just go on. I will have to admit, however, that it was a terrible shock to me when the first one died!

Someone told me recently about an evangelist in the healing ministry years ago who said, "If I prayed for 500, and 500 dropped dead, I'd still go on praying and believing for the sick!!" We feel exactly the same way!

I want to show you another area of persistence, to point out that sometimes we do not understand in the beginning why we are so persistent. Yet, some fifty years down the line we will know.

When I was a young girl growing up, a skinny little Spaniard came into our school auditorium, and he had a machine called a typewriter. Today, everyone is familiar with typewriters, but when I was growing up, a typewriter was really something that very few people had ever seen. He sat down at this machine and it spelled words right out on a piece of paper as plain as anything. He typed 125 words a minute, and I was completely fascinated. My own handwriting was miserable, so I thought a typewriter would be a perfect answer for me, and I purposed in my heart that I was going to be a good typist.

I signed up for a typing class in school. After the first week, I decided it was harder than it looked when he did it, but I had made up my mind that I was going to learn how to type, even though I didn't get up to 125 words per minute the first week.

I went to my teacher and said: "Do you stay after school for a while, and if so, may I stay with you and practice on the typewriter until you go home?"

Then listen to what I said, and it involved a Christian principle I knew nothing about, because I said to her, "I want to practice, because I am going to be the best and the fastest typist that this school has ever seen." I didn't even know what I was talking about, and I could not even hit two keys without making a mistake. But I made that statement because I had purposed in my heart that I was going to be the best typist that the school had ever seen. While the other kids were down at the corner having cokes and cigarettes and doing all the other things that high school kids did at that time, I was sitting in the high school going type, type, type, type, learning how to type!

That wasn't enough, however, because the teacher did not stay long enough after school. We had department stores in St. Louis where I was raised, and so I would spend a dime to get on the bus and go downtown where they had three department stores right in a row.

I would walk into the first one where they had three different typewriters on display and say, "I am interested in typewriters, may I try this one?" I didn't think I was being dishonest, because I didn't say I was interested in buying one, I just said I was interested in typewriters. I would stand there and type on each of the three typewriters until I had the paper completely filled up, then I would thank the clerk and go on to the second store. I would do the same thing there, and then on to the third store. Then I would go back the next day and do the same thing over again!

What I am trying to instill in you is a desire to develop your persistence. I used all the time I could at school! I used all the time after school that the teacher would give me! Then I went to the department stores, and I used up all their paper!

Finally, came the great day when I had my first speed test. If I remember correctly, I typed 31 words a minute with 97 errors! You never saw so many errors in your entire life! Thirty-one words a minute is not bad for a beginner, but 97 errors was absolutely unbelievable! But I purposed in my heart that I was going to be the school's best typist, so I started back on the same routine again. First I would stay after school, then down to the department stores I would go.

Finally the day came when I passed a test at 40 wpm, 50 wpm, 60 wpm, 70 wpm, 80 wpm, 90 wpm, and even 100 wpm, BUT THAT WAS NOT GOOD ENOUGH! I had purposed in my heart that I was going to type 125 wpm like that skinny little Spaniard did! And I wasn't going to settle for less than that, so I kept practicing and practicing until the day came when I typed 125 wpm on a manual typewriter. You really have to put forth energy to type that fast on a manual typewriter. But I did it without any errors whatsoever in a fifteen-minute test! That is what persistence does for you!

I had no more talent in that area than anybody, but I did have persistence! If you keep saying, "I am going to be the world's most dynamic evangelist! I am going to have the world's greatest healing ministry!" do you know what you are going to have? You are going to have exactly what you say, providing you live the life God says! If you will keep on being persistent, and you will keep on doing, even at times when you would like to be doing something else, you will succeed. Be persistent in whatever you do!

At that time I didn't understand why I was learning to type, because most girls want to get married and have a family and never think they are going to use the skills they learn. Little did I realize that my husband was going to die at a very early age, and that I would be thrust out into the business world to raise two children. I praise God for that ability I had because it allowed me to support my children. I owned and operated a secretarial service which eventually turned into a big printing company, but I don't believe that is the only reason God had me learn to type. I don't believe that is why God kept prodding me long before I was a Christian.

Do you know what I think God was doing? God knew that he called me to be an author. God knew that I would have no time to try to write a manuscript in longhand. Fifty years before I ever used the talent, God taught me how to be an oustanding typist, and today I am one of the few authors who type all of their own manuscripts. I do all of my own typing, and after I edit the book I retype it myself, because I know how I like to paragraph, and I know how I like things spaced. I know how I want everything in a book, and these are things I could never have done if I had not been persistent in learning to type.

Now let's get back to Elijah and Elisha. Continuing with II Kings 2, we read in verses 7 and 8 that *"fifty men of the sons of the prophets went, and stood to view afar off: and they two stood by Jordan. And Elijah took his mantle, and wrapped it together, and smote the waters, and they were divided hither and thither, so that they two went over on dry ground."*

Elisha was very impressed with that, so remember it!

Verse 9 says, *"And it came to pass, when they were gone over, that Elijah said unto Elisha, Ask what I shall do for thee, before I be taken away from thee. And Elisha said, I pray thee, let a double portion of thy spirit be upon me."* He wasn't satisfied to have a little crumb of Elijah's power; he wasn't even satisfied to have as much as Elijah; he was a spiritual pig! A spiritual hog! He wanted twice as much! And that is what EACH one of us ought to be — A REAL SPIRITUAL PIG! I love Elisha because he wanted everything God had for him!

Let's watch what Elijah said: *"Thou hast asked a hard thing: nevertheless, if thou see me when I am taken from thee, it shall be so unto thee; but if not, it shall not be so."* I want you to circle the word SEE in this book right now, because it's going to play an important part in your life.

"And it came to pass, as they still went on, and talked, that, behold, there appeared a chariot of fire, and horses of fire, and parted them both asunder; and Elijah went up by a whirlwind into heaven. And Elisha SAW it, and he cried, My father, my father, the chariot of Israel, and the horsemen thereof. And he saw him no more: and he took hold of his own clothes, and rent them in two pieces."

Elisha could have let his attention be distracted by a lot of things. He could have thought, "WOW, look at those trees today, those leaves are really turning." He was a young man, so he could have kept his eyes on girls and missed God! But because he was a persistent man, and he kept his eyes on Elijah, he SAW Elijah when he departed in the whirlwind! AND HE GOT WHAT HE WANTED!

He was a real man of action, because here is faith in action, *"And he took the mantle of Elijah that fell from him, and smote the waters, and said, Where is the Lord God of Elijah? and when he also had smitten the waters, they parted hither and thither: and Elisha went over."*

Elisha could have picked up that mantle and said, "This is so holy and so righteous, I can't put it on." But he knew that God was no respecter of persons, so he picked it up and did the same thing that Elijah did. He thought, "Boy, I will crack that water, and watch that water split open." "POW!" There the waters went! Elisha SAW him when he departed, and then he immediately put into practice what he had seen Elijah do.

I was teaching about persistence on the radio one day, and as I began to teach on this, I suddenly saw a whole new dimension open up through the word "see." I began to think, "Lord, have we been missing out on things because we are not looking with spiritual eyes the way we ought to look?"

A couple of years ago, an evangelist got up in a meeting one night and said, "I had a man come up to me the other night in a meeting, and he handed me a little piece of paper, and he said, 'Brother, the Lord told me to give this to you,' and I thought it was a little note or something." He stuck it in his pocket, thinking it was a prayer request.

He forgot all about it until he got home, and then he took it out of his pocket, and it was a check for $100,000. I always get excited when another ministry receives a big gift, because we rejoice for all ministers of the gospel. WE ARE FOR EVERY CHRISTIAN MINISTRY THAT PREACHES THE GOSPEL OF THE LORD JESUS CHRIST! Neither of us has a jealous bone in our body. I get excited because I always feel that if God does it for one, he will do it for another, since he is no respecter of persons!

Charles and I were driving to a meeting one night and I said, "How come nobody ever walks up to me and says 'Frances, the Lord told me to give you this check for $100,000!'" I was really talking to God, and God said, "Because you never SAW it."

What a surprise that was to me! And I began to think about what he had said! I discovered there are two kinds of visions. There is a supernatural vision which is the kind that God gives you for a particular circumstance and time. And then there is the natural vision where you can stand on the Word of God and begin to see a promise in your spirit, and it will come to pass.

I believe we are in the days of Acts 2:17: *"And it shall come to pass in the last days, saith God, I will pour out of my Spirit upon all flesh: and your sons and your daughters shall prophesy, and your young men shall see visions, and your old men shall dream dreams* (KJV). We all need to be more sensitive to the spirit of God than ever before and to be aware of the part that visions and dreams will be playing in our lives from now on.

In his book, THE FOURTH DIMENSION, Dr. Paul Yonggi Cho says: "Let the Holy Spirit come and quicken the scriptures you read, and implant visions in the young and dreams in the old." In another chapter he says, "... the Holy Spirit comes to cooperate with us — to create, by helping young men to see visions, and old men to dream dreams. Through envisioning and dreaming dreams we can kick away the wall of limitations and can stretch out to the universe. That is the reason that God's word says, *'Where there is no vision the people perish.'* If you have no vision, you are not being creative; and if you stop being creative, then you are going to perish.

"Visions and dreams are the language of the fourth dimension, and the Holy Spirit communicates through them. Only through a vision and a dream can you visualize and dream bigger churches. You can visualize a new mission field; you can visualize the increase of your church."

The vision has to be given to you by the Holy Spirit, or it will not come to pass, because you cannot use your imagination to conjure up things that are not in line with God's Word! But begin to envision according to God's Word, and see what happens!

I quickly turned to Luke 6:38 which says, *"Give, and it shall be given unto you; good measure, pressed down, and shaken together, and running over, shall men give into your bosom. For with the same measure that ye mete withal it shall be measured to you again."*

I said, "Now, Father, Charles and I have given and given and given, and given, and given, and now I think it is time for us to receive a return, because we have so many needs at the City of Light. Father, I am going to ask you to give me a vision of a check."

I must not have had $100,000 faith, because instantly God gave me a vision, but the vision was of a check for $1,000, and all I saw was a man's hand giving it to me.

WOW! Two scriptures, *"my people perish for lack of knowledge"* and *"without a vision the people perish,"* came into my mind. Here I was sitting in a car with a vision of a $1,000 check. That was not unscriptural, because I could stand on Luke 6:38 and KNOW that we had given!

I was so excited I almost ran to get into the meeting that night, and I kept thinking, "Who is it, Lord? Who is it?" I would look at every person who came by and think "You?" "No!" "You?" "No!" "You?" "No!"

Nobody handed me a check that first night.

I didn't say, "I guess God didn't want me to have a check." I am persistent! The second night came and when the service was over, I was standing back at the book table, and every time a man came by, I would think again, "You?" "No!" "You?" "No!" "You?" "No!"

The second night was over, and NOBODY HAD GIVEN ME A CHECK!

I wasn't discouraged, because we still had one more night! I repeated the same procedure, and still no check! I wasn't discouraged, however, and as I was packing the books for the next stop, and in a most unspiritual position of almost standing on my head trying to reach a box, a man walked up behind me and said, "Frances, the Lord told me to give this to you." Hallelujah! I didn't put it in my pocket! I LOOKED AT IT! Right on the spot! IT WAS EXACTLY AS I HAD SEEN IT IN MY SPIRIT — A CHECK FOR $1,000! I nearly exploded!!

I could hardly wait to tell Charles and the next day I was so wound up because I saw a new dimension opening up in our lives, so I said, "Charles this is so exciting, I'm going to ask God for another vision." And I saw another $1,000 check! My faith had not risen any higher than $1,000, but sure enough, about two nights later, a man sent his child running down the aisle before the service started with a check for $1,000. Do you know why? He had given $1,000 the year before and had gotten back over $100,000, so he couldn't wait for offering time to get started again!

Again, I saw a new dimension working! God opening spirit eyes to see more of what he has for us! I was really excited, but I said, "God, could you let me have a little bigger vision? It takes a lot of $1,000 checks to reach the multitudes you have laid on our hearts.

On our next trip, we were leaving our motel room to go to a meeting, when there flashed in my mind a check for $5,000. I thought, "Wow! We have never had anyone put a check for $5,000 into an offering before." But I was excited. I said, "Lord, you mean that you are going to put a $5,000 check in the offering tonight?" And somehow in that way that I know that God speaks, God just assured me that the check was going to be in the offering.

No one ever put that much in one of our offerings before! Nobody! Glory, what a feeling of anticipation we had!

Charles was teaching that night, and after I took the offering, I looked for a place to sit until the ministering time came. The air conditioner had broken down, and the television lights were extremely hot, and I saw a door, so I thought, "I'll go off-stage because it's so hot, and when Charles needs me, I'll come back on."

I stepped off the stage, and discovered that I was in

the room where the ushers were counting the offering. They said, "Would you like to help us count the offering?" My heart was really pounding, because the first thing I did was to try to pull out all the checks. I looked carefully at each one, but there was no check for $5,000.

The ushers were counting the cash when suddenly I saw one more little piece of paper underneath all the bills, and I grabbed for it! You never saw anyone go into action so fast in your life. I opened it up, and it was a check to our ministry for $5,000, THE FIRST TIME IN ALL OF OUR MINISTRY THAT ANYONE HAD EVER PUT IN A CHECK THAT SIZE IN AN OFFERING, JUST AS I HAD SEEN IT! Hallelujah!

Today I see in my spirit a check for $1,000,000 for the work of the ministry. I have confessed it for almost three years! I have seen it in my spirit, and I know it will come to pass!

As a result of seeing in my spirit, I began to think, "If it works in money, why shouldn't it work in other areas as well?" I began to think this should work in the area of healing. I gave this talk about seeing, and then said:

"God made a package deal for us 2,000 years ago, but the problem is that most of us only accept one portion of that package when we are born again, because we don't understand there's more than one 'goodie' in the basket!

"When all churches begin to preach the FULL meaning of salvation, you're going to see people walk into services unsaved, sick, and full of demons, and they are going to walk out saved, healed, delivered, and baptized with the Holy Spirit ALL AT THE SAME TIME!

"Many people believe that salvation involves just one thing: eternal life! Biblically, however, salvation encompasses many things, of which eternal life is only ONE! The Greek word *soteria*, which we translate 'salvation,' also includes the meanings 'deliverance,' 'health,' 'rescue,' and 'safety.'

I continued and said, "How many of you believe that Jesus took all of our diseases on himself at Calvary? Every one of those 39 stripes he had on his back was a different disease."

I believe when Jesus was on the cross that he was the most unhuman looking thing you ever saw. I believe his body was so racked with pain that you would not even have recognized him to be a human being, because can you imagine all of the cerebral palsy from the first man to the last man on the body of Jesus? See him with all the cancer in the world from the first man to the last one.

Every case of diabetes from the first man to the last was on the body of Jesus! Name any disease, and it was on the body of Jesus! Every case of it from the first man to the last man.

I do not believe that Jesus appeared on the cross as most artists paint him. I believe he didn't even resemble the Jesus who had walked up the road to Golgotha!

Isaiah 52:14 (Amp.) says: *"(For many the servant of God became an object of horror; many were astonished.) His face and His whole appearance were marred more than any man's, and His form beyond that of the sons of men; but just as many were astonished at Him."*

Now, why were they astonished when they looked at him? Because his body looked so terrible! Can you imagine all the brain damage in the world on him? Can you see all the crippling diseases on him? Millions of all kinds of diseases, all on Jesus at one time!

Do you think his fingers were straight? No, I think his body was so twisted that we would never have recognized it. That is why they said it was an object of horror, and his face and his whole appearance were marred more than any man's because no other man has ever taken as much on his body as Jesus!

Then it says in Isaiah 53:10: *"Yet it was the will of the Lord to bruise Him; He has put Him to grief and made Him sick . . ."* It was God's will to make him sick! Why? Because he loved you and me so much that he put it on Jesus so that we do not have to have sickness!

Isaiah 53:5 says, *"But He was wounded for our transgressions, He was bruised for our guilt and iniquities: the chastisement needful to obtain peace and well-being for us was upon Him, and with the stripes that wounded Him we are healed and made whole."* WE ARE HEALED AND MADE WHOLE!

Do you know why some of us cannot receive the healing we need? Because we cannot see it on Jesus. I believe the day when our spirit eyes are opened and we begin to see our healing back on Jesus where it belongs is the day you and I are going to receive whatever healing we need! When we begin to see our disease back on Jesus where it belongs, healing will become a reality in our lives!

Begin to see it for yourself. Begin to see it for other people. When you begin to see it, it is going to come to pass in your life. You begin to see your crippled body back on the body of Jesus and that body will be made whole!

But be persistent! If you do not receive healing the first time you "think" you see your disease on Jesus, keep trying! Keep seeing your disease back on Jesus where it belongs! I have a little note in my Bible which says, "He took it, so there's no sense in both of us having it!"

The first night I gave this talk, believing for people to see their diseases back on Jesus I said very carefully, "If there is anybody in the audience who can see their sickness back on Jesus, I want you to come forward." It was a very tense moment for me because I knew I was venturing into a new realm of healing. A man came forward and I said, "What is your problem?" He said, "I was in an industrial accident some fourteen or fifteen years ago. My shoulder blade is frozen, and I can't raise my arm, but as you were talking tonight, I began to see this on Jesus, and before long I saw Jesus with a frozen shoulder. Then I saw myself swinging my arm like I was throwing a baseball, and I haven't been able to move it for 14 years!" All the time he was telling me this, he put his faith into action and was swinging his arm the very way he told me he had seen in his vision! Glory, it was working in healing as well!

Another woman got excited when she saw him, because she had the same problem, and her arm was totally healed that night.

Our faith was really rising in this area of healing, so I gave this talk in another city and began to see what it was doing to people and how their spirit eyes were being opened. Again I gave the same invitation and was very careful to say, "At this time I only want those who have actually seen their problem back on Jesus to come forward!"

I asked the first woman what she saw, and she said, "I see my esophagus full of holes. I see my body full of arthritis. I've got it in the elbows, in the knees, in the hips, and all over me." Do you know what she received? Nothing, because she did not see it on Jesus. She saw it on herself. She was looking at things in the natural. She was not looking at them on Jesus.

The next woman was in a wheel chair. I said, "Honey, what do you see?" She said, 'I see myself walking all the way across this stage tonight." I said, "You do?" She said, "Yes." I said, "How long has it been since you walked?"

She said, "I have never walked. I had polio when I was an infant and I have never walked!"

My faith was really on the line! But I believe that with God nothing is impossible!

She continued, "I see my polio on the body of Jesus!"

Then, just like Elijah said unto Elisha, I said, "If you have seen it on Jesus, it shall be so unto thee." Then I gave her the scripture I always give, *"Silver and gold have I none; but such as I have, give I thee: In the name of Jesus Christ of Nazareth rise up and walk"* (Acts 3:6).

SHE GOT UP AND WALKED, because she saw that she did not have polio any more because it was back on Jesus 2,000 years ago where it belonged. She did not walk like you or I do, but she was walking! Legs that had never moved from the time she was a tiny infant were walking and taking steps across an auditorium!

By this time, my faith really went up, and I was ready to become a tiger. I knew that anyone who could see whatever their disease was back on Jesus Christ would be healed!

A woman in her eighties who was horribly crippled with rheumatoid arthritis came into one of our meetings where I gave this same talk, and I wanted to shake the very devil out of her that caused the horrible arthritis. She was the first one up at the end of the talk, and her crippled fingers straightened out, her back straightened out, and every bit of that rheumatoid arthritis left her! She bent over and touched her toes with her fingers. Glory to God, she had truly seen it back on the body of Jesus where it belonged! In that same service we saw a Catholic man who was so crippled with arthritis that it had been years since he could tie and untie his shoes. He sat on the front row tying and untying his shoes demonstrating that he saw his disease back on Jesus!

We were privileged to be the pacesetter speakers at the Pittsburgh Charismatic Conference one year, and sensitivity to the Holy Spirit really brought results. Sometimes it will go so against your natural mind that it will be almost impossible for you to act, but DO IT!

A woman came over to me prior to the beginning of the service and said, "My daughter is dying. She has been in intensive care for four months. The doctors said she could not even live until the end of the service, but I brought her anyway. Will you come and pray for her?"

Normally I would have taken off like a rocket, but God checked me and said, "Give her the Word first!" Remember what it says in Psalm 107:20, *"He sent his word and healed them and delivered them from their destruction."*

We could not see this girl because we were sitting below stage level, so when we went on to the stage, I saw her for the first time. My first thought was, "Oh, God, don't let her die during this service." I never saw anyone who looked so dead without being dead in my whole life! Her head was hanging over to the side and her tongue was hanging out of her mouth.

Charles took one look at her and thought she had died. He said, "God, is the miracle you want tonight to have us raise someone from the dead?" We have never raised anyone from the dead YET, but we are ready.

All throughout the service I looked at this woman. Her head never changed positions. She never opened her eyes. Nothing, absolutely nothing happened! But when I finished talking about, "If you see it, it shall be so unto you," God said, "Go down and minister to her NOW!"

As Charles and I walked down to this woman, everyone at the conference stood to their feet, wondering what was going to happen! I walked over to this woman and said, "Did you hear what I said?"

A little voice came back to me and said, "Uh huh."

I said, "Did you UNDERSTAND what I said?"

The same little weak voice answered, "Uh huh!"

I said, "What do you see?"

She said, "I see myself completely healed tonight and my disease back on Jesus!" (Note she put a time limit on it!)

I said, "Elijah said, 'If you see me when I go, it shall be so unto thee, but if not, it shall not be so,' so I am

believing that you have seen your disease back on Jesus."
Once again I said, "Silver and gold have I none, but
such as I have, give I thee: In the name of Jesus Christ
of Nazareth, rise up and walk!"

She shot out of that wheel chair full of the power of
God, and walked all the way down the long aisle of the
Duquesne University ballroom with Charles. They
walked all the way down and all the way back.

This woman had been in the intensive care section
of the hospital because she had been hemorrhaging for
four months. The doctors said she would die before the
end of the service because she was in such bad condition, and here she was walking up and down the aisle
of the ballroom having a ball!

The next day she was running all over the mountains where Duquesne University is located saying, "I
don't even feel weak!"

SHE SAW HER SICKNESS BACK ON THE
BODY OF JESUS!

Miracles happen when we can see our problems
back on Jesus who took them all for us!

We went on to another city where we were on a
circular stage. A woman was brought forward who had
multiple sclerosis. I said to her, "What do you see?"

She said, "I see myself healed of multiple sclerosis
because it's on the body of Jesus, and do you know what
else I see?"

I said, "No, what do you see?"

She said, "I see myself running in circles on this big
stage."

I repeated what Elijah said, "If you see me when I
go, it shall be so unto you. You have seen it in your
spirit, now let us see it in the natural."

This woman began running in circles around the
stage. I held her arm, but she almost shook my hand off
saying, "I saw myself running with no help!" Glory,
hallelujah, she didn't run around that circular stage

once or twice, but she must have run around it at least ten times. Why? Because she went into a new dimension, and she saw the sickness where it belonged, back on the body of Jesus Christ!

I could write a complete book on people who have received healing by seeing their sickness back on Jesus, but I believe we can go into the world beyond in many other areas. I think of Pastor Cho when he preached to empty seats, but he never saw one. He preached with his eyes closed, and saw every seat filled. He saw a 10,000 seat auditorium filled to overflowing with people, but if he had opened his eyes, do you know what he would have seen? Maybe 15, maybe 20, maybe 30 or 35 as it grew. He kept his eyes shut. He began seeing in his spirit that great auditorium filled to capacity. Today he has a church with 150,000 members and is seeing in his spirit a church of 500,000! I believe that would never have happened if Pastor Cho had opened his eyes and thought, "Oh, there are only 15 people in the sanctuary today." He closed his eyes instead and saw in his spirit. He saw an auditorium overflowing with people. He saw an auditorium with people standing. He didn't see what was actually there, because he envisioned the lost coming to Jesus in unprecedented numbers! Glory!

I want to emphasize that when I talk about SEE-ING, I am not talking about imagination, but about having faith that a thing will be so! Imaginations can get you into trouble, but a faith vision can bring you answers!

At the City of Light which we are building, God has given us a vision. I can see the world's greatest orchestra at the City of Light. I see God bringing in musicians from all over the country to play at the City of Light. Right now we certainly don't have it, but I know it will be a reality, because I have seen it with my spirit eyes.

I see our School of Ministry overflowing with stu-dents. I see so many students that we won't have enough room for them. That is what I see in my spirit. It is going to come to pass. I believe that with all my heart. I believe it with my soul, and I believe it with my mind!

I believe we will see the glory of God in healing if we will only begin to open up our spirit to see the things God has for us instead of what the devil has for us! Many people find it easier to believe what the devil wants us to see than what God has for us, but it takes a little supernatural vision to look into an area and see what God has for you! The devil wants to see you sick and in poverty, but God said, *"Beloved, I wish above all things that thou mayest prosper and be in health, even as thy soul prospereth"* (III John 2).

If you need healing — see that!

If you need finances — see that!

If you need deliverance — see that!

If you need a mate — see that!

If you need your husband or wife saved — see that!

If you need your children saved — envision them with Bibles under their arms, spreading the gospel!

This is a spiritual and supernatural dimension that can be most rewarding; however, I do want to caution you not to let your imagination get carried away, and don't try to visualize something that you can't line up with God's Word. Line it up with God's Word, and watch it come to pass that WHAT YOU SEE IS WHAT YOU GET!

CHAPTER 8
SOME CONDITIONS FOR HEALING

By Frances

It surprises many people to discover there are conditions to God's healing power! Even so, as you read this, I want you to remember at all times that GOD IS SOVEREIGN!

God can do exactly what he wants to do, exactly when he wants to do it, and he can do it to whomsoever he wills!

Just about the time we think we have everything down pat and know all there is to know about a particular way of healing, do you know what happens? God throws a monkey wrench in the whole thing and says, "Now look, I want to show you that I can do it another way as well!"

However, there are many basic guidelines that we do need to follow, and one is to understand that in many instances there are conditions.

Throughout his Word, God is a God of "our" part and "his" part.

We do our part, and then God does his part.

God says, "You do this, and I'll do that!" Then he says, "You do THIS, and I'll do THAT!"

He is a God of love, a God of mercy, a God of grace: but he puts restrictions on us because we all need rules to go by!

It is the same way with a child. If you brought up a child with absolutely no restrictions whatsoever, you would have a wild little animal of some kind, wouldn't you?

If you let children eat what they wanted to eat, what would they choose? Candy, candy, candy, candy, candy, and that's probably all! But by the time they grew up, they wouldn't have any teeth. They would be very unhealthy; they would not have strong bodies; and so, as parents, we have to bring these children up properly. We need to see that the foods they eat are good for their bodies, so their bodies will not be weak and sickly.

Here's Malachi 4:2 from the Living Bible. *"But for you who fear my name, the Sun of Righteousness will rise with healing in his wings. And you will go free, leaping with joy like calves let out to pasture."*

What is the condition that goes along with that scripture? It is only "for you who FEAR my name!" That is not the kind of fear the devil puts on us. It is the one kind of fear that we all need to have in our lives — the fear and reverence of God. If you want healing in your body, Malachi 4:2 says one condition is to fear the Lord!

There are people in this world today who do not fear the Lord. There are people who curse God until the very end. You might ask, "Doesn't he ever heal a sinner?" Yes, because HE IS SOVEREIGN, he can heal saint and sinner alike!

One night at a miracle rally, an agnostic was sitting in the balcony, making fun of what he thought was nothing but a series of "put-up" healings! Charles pointed up to the balcony and said, "Someone in the balcony has a big lump under his arm. It has been paining you and you have just been healed!" This same man had a tumor the size of a baseball under his arm, and it instantly disappeared! He came running down to the stage as fast as he could and changed his mind about not believing! Miracles will cause a sinner to do a radical turnaround in a hurry!

Proverbs 3:5 says in the Amplified: *"Lean on, trust and be confident in the Lord with all your heart and mind . . ."*

Does it say, "Lean on the Lord with a little bit of you; lean on the Lord on Sunday, but don't worry about Monday, Tuesday and Thursday?" No, it says, *"LEAN ON, TRUST AND BE CONFIDENT IN THE LORD WITH ALL YOUR HEART AND MIND, AND DO NOT RELY ON YOUR OWN INSIGHT OR UNDER-STANDING. In ALL your ways know, recognize and acknowledge Him, and He will direct and make straight and plain your paths. Be not wise in your own eyes; reverently fear and worship the Lord, and turn (entirely) away from evil"* (Prov. 3:5-7 Amp.).

That last verse gives us the conditions, and then verse 8 gives us the reward: *"It shall be health to your nerves and sinews, and marrow and moistening to your bones."* "Learning to Lean" is godly medicine!

If you want your nerves healed, obey the above conditions and see what happens! Best cure I know of!

The last phrase also really speaks plainly to all of us, because it says to turn ENTIRELY away from evil. Not a little bit, but ALL the way!

In the world we live in today, we are beset with temptations every day of our lives! But what does God say? HE SAYS TO TURN ENTIRELY AWAY FROM EVIL!

You cannot live in sin and expect the best from God.

You cannot live over in the devil's workshop a portion of the time, and expect God's abundant life to flow all over you.

You cannot live under the devil's control and expect God's blessings to overtake you and overcome you, because he says to turn entirely away from evil.

Who has to do the turning? WE DO! God doesn't turn you away; God gives you all the power you need; but he leaves it up to you, and he says for YOU to turn entirely away from evil.

There's the condition, and there's the promise. If all the "nervous wrecks" in the world would just lean on, trust in and rely on God, and fulfill the rest of that scripture, we would have fewer nervous wrecks.

What if you were a sinner and you just got saved? Would you have to get healthy before you could become a Christian? No, but sometimes you have to become a Christian before you can get healthy!

Before I was saved, I took nineteen grains of thyroid every day. The doctor told me that I took more thyroid than any person in medical history had ever taken previously. It had been given to me in an attempt to correct an adrenal insufficiency in my body.

I was a victim of Addison's disease and by three o'clock in the afternoon I didn't even look like a human being. My skin would turn so gray it was almost black, and then I would pass out!

God dealt with me one day in a hospital, and I began to seek him, even though I had difficulty admitting that I was a sinner. Nine months rolled around before I was saved; but when I did get saved, I knew that I wanted everything God had for me. I wanted to lean on him, trust him, rely on him, and I certainly wanted to turn away from every evil thing I knew.

God saw my heart, and the day I got saved he healed me instantly! I never took another grain of thyroid from the day I was saved because the healing power of God went through my body, and I was totally and instantly healed of Addison's disease, which is normally fatal. I didn't even realize it until weeks later when I remembered I hadn't taken any medicine!

You may wonder why they gave me thyroid instead of cortisone because this was unusual in treating Addison's disease! The doctors said my thyroid was destroyed because of overdosing me with cortisone; therefore the super doses of thyroid were prescribed. In spite of this, today I have a perfectly normal thyroid gland! Glory to God!

Let's look at another conditional promise. This one is found in Psalm 128 (TLB): *Blessings on all who reverence and trust the Lord — ON ALL WHO OBEY HIM!"* Did you know you can trust and reverence the Lord and still be disobedient? Yes, you can! I know people who go to worship services and say, "Hallelujah, Lord, I bless you; Lord, I praise you," and then walk out the door of the church and right back into sin. A lot of people do that, without even realizing what they are doing. But the Bible says, "Blessings on all who reverence and trust the Lord — on all who OBEY him!" Healing is one of those blessings.

God has a lot of natural laws. There is a time to stay awake, and there is a time to go to sleep. There is a time for everything. God expects you to take care of your body. If you want to stay healthy, don't think that you can stay up night after night without getting sick or run down. I need eight hours of sleep — some people need a little more, some need a little less. But you cannot disregard God's health laws and maintain a healthy body.

There is a price you have to pay if you do! I smoked for 35 years, and ended up smoking five packages a day! Your body suffers when you smoke that many years: it's the worst thing in the world for your circulatory system. Many people die of lung cancer and many die of hardening of the arteries because they have not taken care of their bodies; they have gone on smoking, smoking, smoking, regardless of what God and the government say about how harmful it is. Now that's silly, isn't it? That's just like taking a knife and cutting your throat a little bit each day. Pretty soon you'll have your whole head cut off!

In the Living Bible, Psalm 128 goes on to say, *"Their reward for obeying the Lord will be prosperity and happiness!*" Your reward for obeying the Lord will be prosperity and happiness! It even gives you some specifics: *"Your wife shall be contented in your home. And look at all those children! There they sit around the dinner table as vigorous and healthy as young olive trees. That is God's reward to those who reverence and trust him."*

I love what the Bible says in Hebrews 11:6, *"But without faith it is impossible to please him: for he that cometh to God must believe that he is, and that he is a rewarder of them that diligently seek him."* God gives rewards to those who believe and trust him. GOD IS A REWARDER! I believe that divine health is one of the rewards that God will give you when you diligently seek him. I believe that healing is one of those blessings that come to people who diligently seek him. There is more, too!

He is going to reward you with happiness.

He is going to reward you with abundant life.

He is going to reward you with finances.

He is going to reward you with a good-looking wife or husband!

Healing and health are two of the most important things we could ever desire. If you had to choose between being healthy and being wealthy, it would be far more important to be healthy. It would do you no good at all to have all the money in the world, if you were always in pain.

In the 28th chapter of Deuteronomy, God teaches us many of his conditions for obtaining divine health. In the Amplified, the first condition listed is, *"If you will listen diligently to the voice of the Lord your God."*

To "listen diligently" means to listen with your mind, your heart, your body, your soul, with EVERYTHING you've got! And it doesn't mean listening to God while you're listening to the TV, listening to the radio, and listening to somebody else at the same time. It means that when you listen to God you shut everything else out and just listen to God Almighty, because sometimes God says things that are very soft and very quiet!

The second part of the condition given in Deuteronomy 28:1 (Amp.) is, *"Being watchful to do all His commandments which I command you this day."* It won't do you very much good if you listen to God but don't do what he says! This ties back with the other verse that lists all those blessings which come to those who obey him.

If you are watchful to do all his commandments which I command you this day, Moses says, *"the Lord your God will set you high above all the nations of the earth, And all these blessings shall come upon you and overtake you."*

You have to listen to the voice of the Lord your God, and then you've got to be a doer of the Word and not just a hearer only.

There are many people who run from one meeting to another, from one charismatic conference to another, from one full gospel meeting to another, from one church to another, from one special speaker to another, and who never get out to do a thing they have learned!

I hope one of the things this book will teach you is to quit being a conference hopper and get out there and do something for the Lord: that is one of the ways his blessings of healing and health will come upon you.

Let's look at a similar passage in Isaiah. Here's Isaiah 58:6,7 in The Living Bible: *"No, the kind of fast I want is that you stop oppressing those who work for you and treat them fairly and give them what they earn. I want you to share your food with the hungry and bring right into your own homes those who are helpless, poor and destitute. Clothe those who are cold and don't hide from relatives who need your help. If you do these things, God will shed his own glorious light upon you. He will heal you; your godliness will lead you forward, and goodness will be a shield before you, and the glory of the*

Lord will protect you from behind." GOD WILL HEAL YOU! He will heal you if you live the kind of life he calls us to live.

Here's another familiar passage that stresses this same point: *"If you will diligently hearken to the voice of the Lord your God, and will do what is right in His sight, and will listen to and obey His commandments and keep all His statutes, I will put none of the diseases upon you which I brought upon the Egyptians; for I am the Lord Who heals you"* (Exodus 15:26 Amp.). Here again God is telling us that we need to listen to him and we need to obey him.

Another very well-known passage, Malachi 3:10 says: *"Bring ye all the tithes into the storehouse, that there may be meat in mine house, and prove me now herewith, saith the Lord of hosts, if I will not open you the windows of heaven, and pour you out a blessing, that there shall not be room enough to receive it."*

We hear that verse over and over again. But look at the verse that follows it, because it is the one that tells you what happens when you do what Malachi 3:10 says. It says, *"And I will rebuke the devourer for your sakes, and he shall not destroy the fruits of your ground; neither shall your vine cast her fruit before the time in the field, saith the Lord of hosts."*

There is a blessing promise for many in that verse! Let me show you what I mean. Several years ago a pastor came up to me at the end of a service and said, "We have a missionary family here with two children who have muscular dystrophy. They want you to pray for them."

Muscular dystrophy is an incurable disease which destroys all the muscles and it is generally fatal. We believe that an incurable disease is caused by a spirit, so when we come across an incurable disease, we know the spirit needs to be cast out.

Normally I would have cast out the spirit of

muscular dystrophy, but God said something to me before I started. He said, "Ask them if they tithe!" Wow! That is a difficult question to ask in a church where there were probably 1200 people listening to every word I said. It takes real courage to ask a missionary a question like that where everyone will hear the answer, but God had said, "Ask them if they tithe."

With fear and trembling before the Lord, I said, "Brother, before I lay hands on your children, may I ask you a question?"

"Yes," he answered.

I said, "Do you tithe?"

"I have tithed ever since I became a Christian," he told us.

"Hallelujah!" I said, "Then I will stand on Malachi 3:11, which is a verse so many people forget about, and 'I will rebuke the devourer for your sakes, and he shall not destroy the fruits of your ground; NEITHER SHALL YOUR VINE CAST HER FRUIT BEFORE THE TIME IN THE FIELD, SAITH THE LORD.'

I said, "God is not going to let your vine cast her fruit, he is not going to let your children die before their time. Because you have tithed and you have been faithful to God in your giving, I lay hands on these children and speak healing in the name of Jesus." Then I cast out the spirit of muscular dystrophy. I did not see any visible evidence of healing at that moment but the next morning his little girl got out of bed all by herself for the first time in years and went "leaping with joy like calves let out to pasture." Hallelujah!

Why did that man's children receive healing? Because he had been faithful in his giving to God and God is a rewarder of them who diligently seek him! What joy there was in their hearts because obedience had brought rewards!

There are many different ways to heal, and many different conditions to meet, but keep in mind that God is sovereign; God can do anything he wants to. He can override every single one of the conditions I have mentioned.

Have you ever thought when you saw a rotten, stinking sinner get healed, "Well, God, they never gave you a nickel in their whole life; they're rotten, they don't love you, they even use your name in vain — and you healed them!" Have you ever questioned God about something like that?

Regardless of how you feel, remember GOD IS SOVEREIGN! He doesn't do it this way because you think he ought to do it this way, he does it HIS way because he is a sovereign God! Let's also remember to seek God — not the healing!

CHAPTER 9
ANOINTING WITH OIL

By Charles

Shortly after Frances and I received the baptism with the Holy Spirit, we were sharing the gospel in Indiana. At that time Frances was the only speaker in our family, and I was the CPA who tagged along with her. She saw to it, though, that I had the opportunity to share a little testimony at each service where she spoke.

At this meeting, I began sharing my usual three-minute testimony, when a heavy anointing of the Holy Spirit fell on me and for about an hour scriptures and threads of gold from the Word of God flowed out of me. The message was so divinely anointed that even little children sat completely spellbound the entire time without moving — it was a supernatural act of God!

Two pulpit chairs were to my left; Frances was in one and the other was empty. The pastor was sitting on the front row of pews with his wife. Frances was amazed as she watched the way God's powerful anointing was changing her husband.

After quite a while, Frances felt the sheer sleeve of her dress move from a light breeze apparently caused by someone sitting down next to her. She assumed it was the pastor who had come up to remind her that he had called her to speak, and not me.

A few more minutes went by, then someone tugged

at her sleeve, so she decided she had better look to see what the pastor wanted. As she turned, she was shocked to discover it wasn't the pastor at all! What she saw sitting next to her, relaxed, with his arms resting on the arms of the chair and his legs crossed, was JESUS!

His form was clearly visible, but he was transparent! A soft but brilliant blue glow surrounded his entire being! Frances said, "I was absolutely overcome with the presence of God! I couldn't take my eyes off of him."

Jesus looked at Frances, then pointed to the bottle of olive oil on the stand next to the pulpit and said, "That is symbolic of the Holy Spirit." Then he pointed to me and said, "That's the real oil! Because the anointing is on him, let Charles speak tonight!" If you will recall, oil in the Old Testament symbolically refers to the Holy Spirit.

After almost an hour of talking, I suddenly stopped speaking and said, "You have come to hear Frances tonight, and I must stop!" so Frances, with the glory of God all over her, quickly stepped to the microphone and told the audience what had just happened and related that Jesus had said Charles was to speak because the anointing was on him!

For a few moments I struggled in the flesh as I began speaking again, but soon the anointing began to flow! What a night it was! After the service, someone in the audience told us that they noticed the struggle I was going through when I was trying to get started again, so they prayed for the anointing to return. They reported that waves of power started at the back row of pews and moved forward, gaining momentum until they reached the pulpit and then fell on me!

What a night of glory and power! One of the men in the congregation left the church around eleven o'clock and went racing up and down the streets of this small town, knocking on doors saying, "The Holy Spirit has fallen! The Holy Spirit has fallen!" Flames of fire were reported to have been seen coming out of his coattails!

Afterwards I began to ponder on the scripture about anointing with oil and praying for the sick. I said, "God, why do we need to use oil, which is only symbolic of the Holy Spirit, when we have received the real Holy Spirit power through the baptism with the Holy Spirit?" James 5:13-15 is in the New Testament, and it was written after the disciples received the baptism with the Holy Spirit.

"Is any sick among you? let him call for the elders of the church; and let them pray over him, anointing him with oil in the name of the Lord: And the prayer of faith shall save the sick, and the Lord shall raise him up; and if he have committed sins, they shall be forgiven him" (James 5:14,15).

I thought, "Jesus, before the day of Pentecost you told your twelve apostles to go out two by two and you gave them power over unclean spirits. They did what you told them to do, and your Word says, *'And they went out, and preached that men should repent. And they cast out many devils, and anointed with oil many that were sick, and healed them'* (Mark 6:12,13).

"Why, Jesus, do we need to anoint with oil to heal the sick if we have the power to do so through the baptism with the Holy Spirit?"

The reason he gave me is this: God loves every Christian equally. He does not love those who have received the baptism with the Holy Spirit any more than he loves the Christians who have not yet received the enduement of power promised. *"And, behold, I send the promise of my Father upon you: but tarry ye in the city of Jerusalem, until ye be endued with power from on high"* (Luke 24:49).

Since he loves us all alike, and wants us to be in health, he has provided a way for healing, other than the Holy Spirit power flowing from a Spirit-filled

Christian into a sick body. Instead he made provisions for those who love and serve him to be able to ask HIM to do the healing.

Jesus said in Mark 16:17,18, *"And these signs shall follow THEM that believe; In my name shall THEY cast out devils; they shall speak with new tongues* (that's the baptism with the Holy Spirit with the evidence of speaking in other tongues); *They shall take up serpents; and if they drink any deadly thing, it shall not hurt them; THEY shall lay hands on the sick, and they shall recover."*

Prayer generally is asking God to do something. Notice in the above scripture that Jesus did not tell us to pray, but he told us to do the healing ourselves by the laying on of hands. We do anoint with oil when asked, because that will also heal the sick, but we personally do not feel it is necessary once you have received the baptism with the Holy Spirit, for the power of God IN you will flow out of your hands into the sick body or mind and that power will do the healing. If you have not received the baptism with the Holy Spirit, the enduement of power, then you have the authority of the Word of God to ASK GOD TO DO THE WORK FOR YOU, and he will!

God's Word can never be limited to our human understanding, so there may be many other ways God uses the anointing with oil in relation to healing the sick. Other meanings than those I have given above may be revealed to you. That's great! Always do what God leads you to do, because God doesn't always do it the way we think it should be done!

"But God hath chosen the foolish things of the world to confound the wise; and God hath chosen the weak things of the world to confound the things which are mighty" (I Cor. 1:27).

Frances loves to tell about a healing where God did seem to use a foolish thing to perform a mighty miracle.

In a small town in Louisiana, some ladies called for

prayer for a friend who had cancer. They had been reading in James that the elders should anoint with oil and pray with faith for healing, so they decided to obey God's Word.

The pastor was out of his office at the time, and there were no elders available either. They decided they should do something, and since there was no one else present, they felt that ought to make them elders. They stopped by the grocery store on the way to pray, and bought a gallon of cooking oil. The lady was in bed, and because the Bible didn't give the exact amount of oil to use when praying for the sick, THEY POURED THE WHOLE GALLON OF OIL ALL OVER THE POOR WOMAN while they were praying the prayer of faith! But God honored their faith, and totally healed the woman of cancer! Glory! We certainly don't recommend a whole gallon of oil, but it certainly brought results in this case.

If you are succeeding in getting the sick healed or delivered another way than what we recommend, praise God, don't slow down or change — keep doing what God has led you to do! However, if you are not getting them all healed, try some of our ways and see if they won't work for you, too!

AND DON'T FORGET — GOD IS SOVEREIGN!

CHAPTER 10
HEALING THROUGH INTERCESSORY PRAYER

By Frances

Do you remember the story in Matthew 8, about the Centurion who said to Jesus, *"Speak the word only, and my servant shall be healed?"* People are healed the same way today! A friend or a relative stands in a prayer line for someone possibly thousands of miles away, and they are healed by the power of God, because God is omnipresent. It is fascinating to realize that God can be everywhere at exactly the same time!

Some years ago, I was invited to a non-charismatic church near Houston. At the end of the service, I began to share what God is doing in the world today, as he pours out his Spirit on all flesh!

I told them I sincerely believe that we are in the very last age; I do not believe there will be another generation beyond us — I believe Jesus will come back long before this generation passes away. So I began to share that this is why I believe we see a greater outpouring of the Spirit of God now than we have ever seen in our entire life.

After the meeting, a woman came up to me and said she had a friend whom the doctors said was dying. She was in intensive care, in a hospital miles away. She said, "Do you believe God would heal her?" I told her that all I know is what the Bible says, and it says that

Jesus told the Centurion, " *'Go thy way; and as thou hast believed, so be it done unto thee.' And his servant was healed that selfsame hour"* (Matt. 8:13).

I thought to myself, "What do I have to lose?" When I lay hands on a sick person, I do not have anything to lose regardless of whether they get healed or not, because the Bible tells me to be dead to self. When you are dead to self, you cannot worry about your reputation. No dead person ever sat up in a casket and complained, "But what about my reputation?"

I began to pray for this woman's friend. I said, "Father, I don't even know who she is. I certainly don't know what her problem is. But, God, I ask you to do the supernatural and go out and touch her and make her every whit whole from the top of her head to the tip of her toes." Then I said, "Thank you." Those words are two of the most important words you will ever say. When you say, "Thank you, Jesus," do you know what you are doing? You are saying, "Jesus, I believe that you did it, so I am going to say, 'Thank you!' " If we REALLY believe that God has heard our prayer, then we are ungrateful if we do not say thank you!

Even if you pray for a thousand people in a prayer line, say thank you after each one. Every time you say thank you, you are telling God "I believe that it is done, and I receive it as a completed miracle in Jesus' name."

After I prayed for the woman's friend, I said, "Thank you, Jesus," but then I did something I had never done previously. I looked at my watch, and said, "It is 11:37." I didn't know at the time why I said it, but I do today!

In a hospital miles away, something else happened at exactly 11:37. Jesus Christ walked into a hospital room! A lady in intensive care who was supposed to be dying of cancer immediately got out of bed! She very carefully took all the needles out of her arm, disconnected the oxygen, walked out into the hospital corridor and went to the head nurse!

The shocked nurse said, "What happened to you?"

The woman said, "Jesus Christ personally came into my room at 11:37 and said, 'Shirley, get out of bed. You are healed.' "

The nurse said, "Did you have a vision?"

Shirley said, "No, Jesus Christ personally walked into my room!"

What a loving Father we have! God's supernatural power had touched her the very instant I prayed, and confirmed it by telling me to look at my watch, so we would know that Jesus went into action in answer to prayer that same instant in a hospital miles away!

Sometimes we may feel it is easier to pray for someone when we can lay hands on them, and see them, but start praying more prayers of intercession for people at distances, and watch the miracles God begins to do.

Make a list right now and get busy praying!

CHAPTER 11
HEALING THROUGH USE OF PRAYER CLOTHS

By Frances

Prayer cloths are another instrument used to heal the sick. So far as I know, the Bible only mentions them once, but God really shouldn't have to tell us any more than that, because if it happened once in the Bible, it can happen again today!

Acts 19:11,12 tells us that *"God wrought special miracles by the hands of Paul: so that from his body were brought unto the sick handkerchiefs or aprons, and the diseases departed from them, and the evil spirits went out of them."*

We often send prayer cloths from our office to people who write and say, "I believe that if you pray over this handkerchief (or send me a prayer cloth), I will be healed."

It is difficult for the natural mind to understand, but there is POWER in a piece of cloth when the anointing of God rests on it! Tremendous unlimited divine power can be contained in anything, so when someone requests a prayer cloth, we send them a little piece of polyester about two inches by two inches. This would mean nothing, except before we mail it out, we lay hands on it, pray over it, and believe God for a miracle!

Because we BELIEVE those little pieces of cloth are anointed, many people have been healed when we have sent them out!

One of the most exciting incidents started when we received a letter from a grandmother in Failsworth, England. She had heard about our healing ministry and wrote us a letter. In it, she told us about her grandbaby who had been born with a congenital hip defect, plus a huge waterhead (hydrocephalus). A waterhead baby rarely lives very long because that is a very serious malformation of the body, strictly from the devil, and certainly not given by God.

"If you can't come to England," she wrote, "Would you please send me a little prayer cloth?"

England is a long way from Houston, Texas, so we and our entire office staff laid hands on a little piece of cloth. We asked God to let his healing power go into it, and along with it, so that when it was laid on the baby, resurrection power would go from the cloth into the baby's body, and the baby would be totally healed by the power of God!

We believed with supernatural faith as we prayed over that little piece of cloth and sent it on its divine road. The baby was asleep when it arrived, so the grandmother took the little piece of cloth, rolled it up and stuck it inside the baby's hand. That was her point of contact!

Grandma wrote and told us that the very second that little prayer cloth touched the inside of the baby's fist, the waterhead instantly reduced to normal size. THAT BABY WAS NO LONGER A WATERHEAD. The child was totally and instantly supernaturally healed by the power of God!

Our letter to that English grandmother had to go all the way across the Atlantic Ocean. Even though it was just in a paper envelope, the anointing of God stayed on the prayer cloth as it went from Houston, probably to New York, and then from New York to London and then on another kind of carrier from London to Failsworth, England. THE POWER OF GOD WAS STILL THERE! Probably a week or ten days elapsed between the time it was prayed over and the time it was put in the hand of that child, but the power had not diminished! That power was as strong as when we prayed, and so was the receptive faith of the grandmother!

Two weeks later they took this child back to the clinic where it had been previously treated, and when the doctor X-rayed the baby's hips, he found two perfect hip sockets. The child had been born without any hip sockets at all, and now it had two! The grandmother related that the doctor at the clinic said, "This is not the same baby we have been treating. The medical records show that the child has no hip sockets. The medical records show that the child has a waterhead. What did you bring this one for? This one has no waterhead and has two hip sockets." Hallelujah!

Prayer cloths can also be used for other things beside healing! While I was teaching about prayer cloths at the City of Light School of Ministry, one of our students stood and asked to share part of her testimony.

"Three years ago," she said, "you gave me a prayer cloth. You told me to go home, put the prayer cloth under my husband's pillow, and believe that he would be saved before the end of the year."

"I put the prayer cloth under my husband's pillow in January, and he was saved in November of that same year."

"Before that time, I hadn't wanted anything to do with prayer cloths, because I used to get letters from certain ministries saying that they would send me a prayer cloth if I would send them an offering."

"That day I realized it was not a piece of cloth that would save my husband, but the anointing of the Holy

Spirit. Praise God, yesterday was the third anniversary of his salvation, and he stood in our church to testify."

PRAYER CLOTHS WORK!

If you have the baptism with the Holy Spirit, lay your hands on some little cloths, and start putting them where they are needed! Many, many husbands have been saved through a prayer cloth under their mattress!

People have written to us who have glued them under the seats of teachers in schools, and they insist this is what has brought about the salvation of the teacher! I never heard anyone talk of putting them under students' chairs, but it might be a good idea!

Also, please remember that you do not need to have some big evangelist lay hands on a prayer cloth. YOU HAVE EXACTLY THE SAME POWER OF GOD.

That is why we are so excited about this book. We can hardly wait to see what is going to happen as a result of what you're reading right now! Get busy!

CHAPTER 12
OTHER WAYS TO HEAL THE SICK

By Frances

Faith in Action

One of the most important things we need to remember at all times is that God does want to heal us. Over and over again in his Word, he tells us about his healing power, and he wants us to appropriate it for today.

Matthew 12:10,13 is an important scripture because it talks about faith in action, which is one of the most important ways to bring about a healing. *"And behold, there was a man which had his hand withered ... Then saith he to the man, Stretch forth thine hand. And he stretched it forth; and it was restored whole, like as the other."*

That was FAITH IN ACTION. Jesus gave him a specific task to do. He was probably sitting there with an undersized, deformed little hand and he could have said, "Jesus, I was born with a withered hand. Can't you see I can't stretch it out?" But he didn't. He did exactly what Jesus told him to do. As he completed his faith in action, that arm was totally made whole!

That same story is told in Mark 3:10-15 and Luke 6:6-10. Exactly the same story, but with the different perspectives of each of the three writers. God could have edited the Bible and taken out anything he wanted to take out, but he repeated it so you would believe those stories were actually true. You will note that there are some scriptures in this book that we have used over and over again so they will stick in your mind and you will remember them!

"When he had thus spoken, (he had just finished telling them that he was the light of the world) *he spat on the ground, and made clay of the spittle, and he anointed the eyes of the blind man with the clay, And said unto him, Go, wash in the pool of Siloam, (which is by interpretation, Sent.) He went his way therefore, and washed, and came seeing"* (John 9:6,7).

When did the miracle occur? Did the miracle occur when Jesus spit? Did the miracle occur when Jesus made the mud pie? Or did it occur when the man put his faith into action?

When did it occur? WHEN HE PUT HIS FAITH INTO ACTION. Jesus could have spit all over the place. Jesus could have made mud pies from here to there, and he could have put them on the eyes of every person there, but I doubt that anybody would have been healed, until they obeyed the command, *"Go, wash in the pool of Siloam."*

That would be a ridiculous command, because the man was blind. How could he find his way down to the pool of Siloam? He had been there lots of times, but not without help. God can always do the supernatural. He can take a blind man right through every street without getting him run over.

The blind man could have said, "It is a long way to Siloam. You can just touch me and I will be healed." He could have said, "I don't know how to get there. I never heard of the place." Or he could have said, "I don't like the smell of the water down there. Smells like sulphur!" He could have used all kinds of excuses, but when he obeyed the command, went down and washed the clay off his eyes, he was healed by the power of God, because he had put his faith into action.

We have told you stories all the way through this book about various people who were healed because they put their faith into action.

The story of Naaman as told in II Kings 5:1-15 is an exciting story of faith in action. The Bible says that Naaman was a great man and honorable, and a mighty man of valour, but he was a leper. The devil will attack anybody. He does not attack just a poor nobody all the time. He goes to the top rank and hits the general and the privates all the way down the line.

There was a little servant girl there whom God used in this great man's life. Most people would have thought a little servant girl was at the bottom of the barrel, but she told Naaman how he could be healed. The person who had the lowest position in the house was the one whom God instructed. As we have said over and over, God is no respecter of persons. He does not care who you are. He just cares whether or not you are available and willing to do what he tells you to do.

Naaman took along a lot of silver and gold because he was going to try and buy his healing, but you cannot buy a healing from God. God's healing is absolutely free. The price was paid 2,000 years ago when Jesus died on the cross! I have a feeling that when Naaman got to the door, he thought Elisha would come out and bow down and say, "Hello, Mr. Bigshot. I am so glad you are here today. I respect the fact that you are a great man and a big general, and you have a lot of money and a lot of chariots!" Elisha didn't even come out to greet him!

Elisha was not being impolite. I believe God was teaching a lesson to Naaman, because Elisha sent a messenger and told him to go wash in the Jordan seven times and that he would be made whole.

Naaman had a big decision to make here. The Jordan River was not nearly as nice as the river that

Naaman had in his own backyard.

What would you think if you had gone with your best outfit on, your very best clothes, the very best of everything you had, and this prophet merely tells you to go down to that muddy river and jump in seven times. Not only one time, but SEVEN TIMES! You might have reacted exactly as Naaman did! He was mad! But praise the Lord for the fact that Naaman had some smart people working under him, and they went on to remind him that if Elisha had told him to do some great thing he would have done it. But Elisha had asked him to do something that was beneath his dignity!

A lot of people have the same problem, but Naaman listened to his friends and went down and dipped himself seven times in the Jordan with all of his good clothes on. Can you imagine the cleaning bill he had when he came out of that muddy river? But he was obedient. Hallelujah, Naaman dipped himself not one time, not two times, not three times, not four times, not five times, not six times, but seven times. YES! There is that perfect number of God!

If Naaman had never done a thing, he would have died a leper, but because he was willing to be obedient, he was willing to humble himself and go down there and dip himself in the muddy water, he was healed by the power of God! He put FAITH INTO ACTION!

Faith is something you must put into action. It is not a stationary thing. There is no neutral in faith. You are either going up or you are going down. Your faith will never stay on the same level. You get into the Word of God every day, and what happens to your faith? It begins to go "up, and up, and up!" You stay out of the Word of God and what happens to your faith? It begins to go "down, and down, and down!" That is why you must put your faith into action. You must read your Bible! Did you know that Bible reading is an "act of action?" It takes stamina, and it takes discipline to get into the Word of God and read the Bible, so we need to keep our faith in action at all times. If you never went out and put your faith in action, and you never went out and put this teaching in action, do you know how much you would accomplish? NOTHING, ABSOLUTELY NOTHING! What will happen when you do? EVERY-THING, EVERYTHING, EVERYTHING!

Under the Power
Some of our greatest healings have occurred while people have been slain by the Spirit of God! One in particular that really thrills our hearts occurred seven years ago.

A young lady had been brought to our meeting from an insane asylum. She had been heavily sedated, but her mother had faith to believe that if we laid hands on her she would be healed!

She knew nothing about the meeting. She was so drugged, her mind could not comprehend anything that was going on, but at the end of the service, the mother brought her forward, and we laid hands on her. She fell under the power of God, and we never saw her again until seven years later.

She told her story like this: "I don't remember a single thing about the meeting. I don't even remember being there. All I remember is waking up while lying on the floor and seeing Jesus with his hands outstretch-ed to me. In that instant I was saved, and then I began to speak in tongues, something I knew nothing about! My mind was completely clear and I have had no problems since that time when I was slain by the Spirit of God, and a miracle happened in my life!" Saved, baptized and healed all at one time! Glory!

After a meeting one night, a president of the Full Gospel Businessmen's Fellowship was taking us to the motel when his wife said, "I got so involved in the service tonight I forgot to go up for healing for myself."

Charles said, "What do you need Jesus to do?"

She said, "I have a spinal bifida caudal which has caused me to have pain all my life. As a matter of fact, my mother used to wrap me in a blanket and put me in the oven to try to alleviate the intense pain."

Charles said, "As soon as we get to the motel, we will lay hands on you."

And that's exactly what we did, right in the lobby of the motel! She fell under the power, and while she was there, her body moved around on the floor, and she said, "I feel like something is happening inside of me!"

When she got up off the floor, she said, "The pain is gone, it's ALL gone!" She said she had felt like something was being added to her body and hooked up while she was on the floor! We have heard from her since then and she is still on a cloud because of how God healed her when she was under the power! THERE IS POWER UNDER THE POWER!

Barren Women

I have that special "faith without a doubt" when someone is barren or incapable of producing a baby. I love to minister in this area, and there are little "Hunter babies" all around the world! I use two scriptures, Psalm 113:9, *"He maketh the barren woman to keep house, and to be a joyful mother of children,"* and Exodus 23:26: *"There shall nothing cast their young, nor be barren, in thy land: the number of thy days I will fulfill."* Our files are full of wonderful miracles about barren couples who have conceived and brought forth healthy children even after years of infertility. Most of the time these couples are slain by the Holy Spirit, and this is when the healing takes place. Glory!

By Charles

Strokes

A man had been paralyzed down his right side for three years; his leg was as stiff as a board and he could not bend his knee at all; his right arm was totally incapable of moving and had been drawn up against his waist with the fist so tightly closed that his hand was white from lack of circulation.

As I started to minister to him, the Spirit of God descended on me so mightily that it was like a warm energy flowing through every cell of my head and shoulders, then God spoke three silent but distinct words into my brain: "SPIRIT OF DEATH!"

I didn't understand all that God meant, but I knew it was God, and I knew that if he said it was a spirit, I was to cast the spirit out. I also knew that Jesus called spirits by what they did. Without taking time to understand, I quickly bound Satan by the power of the Holy Spirit, and commanded the "spirit of death" to come out in the name of Jesus!

Then the "word of wisdom" began to operate, but I didn't realize until later that God was speaking to me by this supernatural gift of the Spirit to show me how to heal stroke victims. I began to minister in a way that was similar to therapy. First I said, "Say, 'Jesus I love you!'"

He repeated my words, but not clearly. His wife was excited about that because previously he could not speak!

Then I took his immobile arm and began to bend it back and forth at the elbow. It was very stiff at first, but began to limber each time I bent it. It was not frozen in place. Soon it was free, and he could move it, slightly at first, but finally nearly normally.

I did the same thing with his leg. Then I began

opening his fist and bending his fingers back and forth. Within about five minutes, he was able to lift his arm and walk bending his leg without any help. Within four days he had almost completely recovered.

At another meeting, we discovered the left side of a woman's face was dead from a stroke. The spirit of death was commanded to come out, and I had her pat her face with her hand for about five minutes. The feeling totally came back into her face.

I could name scores who have been healed in similar ways, and yet some seem not to improve. I personally believe that the environment into which they return has a lot to do with their improvement. If the family or friends express no faith and give no encouragement or aid, they regress if healing has started. If they are with someone who has strong faith and encourages and works with them, I believe tremendous results will occur.

You can heal stroke victims the same way I do! Be patient and loving with them as you minister, but do not sympathize, because sympathy is one of the biggest killers in stroke cases!

I asked a Spirit-filled medical doctor what happens when a person has a stroke. He said usually they have a blood clot in a vessel, or a rupture of the vessel, which keeps the oxygen and food supply from going into a portion of the brain. As a result, the brain cells become dormant or die. Therapy will sometimes bring a dormant cell back to activity.

What I believe now is that when a "spirit of death" is cast out, the spirit which brought about the clot leaves and the flow of blood to the cells restores activity. All you have to do is apply faith and therapy to re-educate the communication between the brain and the paralyzed portion of the body. By bending the arm, leg, and fingers, as well as using the tongue in speaking, the brain begins sending signals and the limbs respond.

There is really nothing wrong with the arm or leg,

but since the brain cell cannot send signals, the arm or leg quits functioning. If you are a doctor or nurse and this isn't described quite right technically, you can still get the idea.

Be careful as you bend a limb, because if the people are not healed you could hurt them. Stroke victims often cry when you talk with them. When you bend a limb, it may hurt, or they may act like it hurts. This requires extreme sensitivity to the Holy Spirit! I generally tell stroke victims that I am going to cast a spirit of pain out and that it will not hurt the next time I bend it. Sometimes I simply rebuke the pain if I feel it is not a spirit. Almost always the pain leaves them.

Hay Fever & Sinus

God healed me of hay fever in 1970, after more than thirty-five years of suffering. This he did supernaturally, but from time to time I had a problem with sinus. Somewhere during the year of 1977, it became so severe I had to take three pills a day plus a shot about every three or four weeks to kill the infection. Finally, after about a year of this with both of us praying night and day for healing I said, "God, please show me how to get rid of this!"

Shortly after this we were in the home of a medical doctor in Florida eating lunch, when the doctor's wife said, "I'm sorry I don't have any coffee or tea to give you, but we all had such severe sinus problems, we all quit drinking coffee and tea and started drinking a lot of juices, and sinus left the entire family within three or four weeks."

I said, "Thank you, Jesus!"

I quit drinking coffee and tea and started drinking all the orange and apple juice my system would take, and within a few weeks the sinus problem was healed!

A singer friend of ours went to a doctor for a prescription for a sinus infection. The doctor gave him a slip and when he looked at what the doctor wrote, he said, "But doctor, I want something to dry this stuff up!" The doctor had prescribed fourteen glasses of water daily! He took the prescription and it worked!

All healing comes from God whether it's under the heading of preventive medicine or common sense! The healings in this particular area seem to be related to possibly plain old common sense!

Mass Healings

Backs, necks and knees are three areas of the body with which a lot of people have problems. When we feel the Spirit leading us to minister in groups, we call everyone forward who has a problem in whatever area the Spirit has revealed to us will be healed at that time. We line them up shoulder to shoulder and then give a word of explanation as to what is going to happen.

We use the principle of laying hands on the sick, and faith in action. We tell them we are going to lay hands on their necks (or knees) and as soon as we do, we ask them to move their necks vigorously as soon as we have touched them. We have often noticed that the healing occurs as soon as their faith goes into action, and we also notice that those who do not move their necks do not receive their healing!

We have seen over one hundred people with neck problems healed at one time! The same thing happens to knees when people put their faith into action! This can happen in almost any type of disease. One night we saw more than two hundred people healed of arthritis all at the same time. A sound came over the auditorium like bones cracking, as the arthritis was healed!

Back problems are in a different category, and we share about that in another chapter.

You may not ever minister to more than one individual at a time, but who knows what God is going to do in the near future in your life — you may be ministering to the masses, so you will need to know how to do that, too!

Some Clues to Success

We hope we have given you some clues as we share the different ways to heal the sick which can help you as an individual with a desire to heal or be healed!

If we asked the typical, average Christian to minister healing to an individual, the first thing he would do would be to close his eyes as tightly as he possibly could. For some reason or other, we try to be "religious," or to impress God in some way with how super-spiritual we are, so here are a few little things to remember:

Being pious won't heal the sick!

Being religious won't heal the sick!

Squeezing your eyes shut won't heal the sick!

Being afraid to minister won't heal the sick!

We haven't healed everyone that we've ministered to, but we see more and more people being healed all the time, so get rid of "self" so that you won't worry about what people think about you, and come along and learn how to heal the sick, IN THE NAME OF JESUS!

BE NATURAL in whatever you do. Be very natural. I have a little "scripture" written in the back of the Bible on the white pages that says: "Keep thy big mouth shut when I pray!"

The reason I say that is because Jesus told us to be in one accord and he said if two or more of us agree as touching anything, it would be done for us. If I am ministering healing to you, God may have a special word of wisdom or a word of knowledge that you need to hear. But if I am laying hands on you, and you are saying, "Oh, Jesus! Oh, Jesus! Thank you, Jesus! Please heal me, Jesus!" you are not hearing a word I am saying. You are not hearing the very word that you need to hear to be healed! Plus the human mind isn't big enough to go in two channels at once. YOU CANNOT TRANSMIT

AND RECEIVE AT THE SAME TIME.

If you are praying and I am praying, how can you possibly agree with me when you don't know what I'm saying? And how can I possibly agree with you when I can't hear you? If you want to praise God and love God, do it every way you can! Praise God in your native language, pray in tongues, call on his name, speak the Word, but when you are being ministered to for healing, just keep your ears tuned in and "keep thy big mouth shut!"

I have a special reason for saying this, because we have noticed that very few people go under the power of God when they are talking or praying in tongues as we lay hands on them. Neither do they get healed! We certainly believe in praising and worshiping God, but it is not timely when you are dividing your attention and not in complete agreement!

We have had individuals come up and say, "There's a severe burning right in my hands, right where the nail went through Jesus' hand, and when that burning comes in, I KNOW I've got the healing power upon me." Let us always remember that Jesus didn't tell us to watch for a burning sensation in our hands, or any special kind of feeling, but he did tell the believer to go out and lay hands on the sick and know they would recover!

Don't ever depend on your feelings alone! There have been many times when we did not "feel" any particular anointing of any kind, and yet we have stood on what the Word of God says, and not our feelings, and great miracles have taken place.

Looking for feelings instead of healings can rob you of what God wants to do through you. Develop compassion, however, and don't ever become legalistic or you'll leave the love of God out! Ask God to give you a special love for those who are sick and hurting!

CHAPTER 13

WHAT IF I DON'T GET HEALED?

By Frances

What do you do when you have done everything you know to do to have faith to be healed? What do you do when it seems that about everyone who has ever been used to heal the sick has already prayed for you, and you're still sick?

What do you do when it seems like all hope is gone and time is running out? What more can you do when you have seemingly already done all that you know to do?

We have seen the percentage of people who get healed in our services increase dramatically over the years. We have learned many ways to heal, and our faith has increased mightily because we have seen God's miracle power work repeatedly as we have used different ways he has shown us to apply his healing power. Yet, our knowledge, understanding, and discernment, and our perfecting of the operation of the abilities given through the Holy Spirit have not reached that of Jesus when he was operating on this earth.

We urge those who don't get healed when we minister to them to have others minister to them because God seems to give special faith to some for a particular healing, and to others faith for healing of different sicknesses. If we minister this year without success, try us again the next time you see us because God may have added new faith or new ways to heal the sick which will succeed for you.

Many years ago I developed an ulcer on my leg due to phlebitis which I acquired during my "smoking" days. I have been prayed for over and over by the "best of them!" I have quoted scriptures and stood on the Word. Charles has commanded; I have commanded. Charles has laid hands on me; I have laid hands on myself. Upon occasion we had whole congregations lay hands on me for healing, and nothing seemed to work.

When we finished the final teaching at the City of Light School of Ministry on how to heal the sick, the devil really took a wild fling at my leg, and I couldn't even stand up! The pain in my leg was so intense I couldn't stand it sitting up, lying down, or standing up! The infection had spread to my entire leg, but in my spirit I felt condemned because that healing would not manifest itself!

I called John Osteen, a beloved brother in Christ, and told him the doctor wanted me in the hospital immediately. He instantly began to pray and said, "Father, let her go to the hospital with no condemnation in her heart. We know that all healing comes from you, and we thank you that YOU are the one who is going to complete this healing, and we thank you in Jesus' name!"

With no feeling of condemnation, I immediately went to the hospital. A bone specialist cut out the diseased tissue, and much to the surprise of everyone, my leg healed in absolutely record time. They had advised me that my stay in the hospital would be for several weeks. Charles had a word of knowledge and told the doctor that I would be out in eight days, and on the eighth day I came out!

As a result of my visit, my hospital roommate

accepted Jesus, her husband and son got saved, and they all three were filled with the Holy Spirit. Even my doctor said, "God has got to be in this!" Hallelujah!

So if you've tried and tried like I did, and nothing seems to work, go without condemnation and seek medical help! I did, and now my leg is fine!

CHAPTER 14

BEING SENSITIVE TO THE HOLY SPIRIT!

By Frances

We don't go through airports or down the street looking for people to heal, because we believe the Holy Spirit will draw people to you whom he has already prepared. We simply minister healing when we have an opportunity, whether it is to one individual or to multitudes; whether it is in a church or on the street.

One time we were in the Atlanta airport, and as we were walking to the gate, I stopped in the ladies' restroom. There was a lady sitting there in a wheel chair, and the Holy Spirit implanted the thought into my mind that I was to minister to her. I certainly do not do this all the time; I just had an impression that I should pray for her.

Months later I received a clipping from a newspaper sent to me by a woman who knew us. Under the headline of SALLY JONES HEALED BY UNKNOWN WOMAN IN ATLANTA AIRPORT, was an article which said something to this effect: Sally Jones, who has been crippled from birth, went into the rest-room in Atlanta on a recent trip. A woman walked up to her and said, "My name is Frances Hunter and I'm a Christian. May I pray for you?"

Sally said, "I'll take all the prayer I can get."

She related that the woman simply laid hands on her and left the room. After the woman had walked out the door, Sally Jones said she realized she was healed, so she got up out of the wheel chair to run and thank her, but the woman had already disappeared into the crowd. Sally has no idea who the woman was, other than her name!

Be sensitive to the leading of the Holy Spirit. Notice that I did not just go up and lay hands on the woman, but I introduced myself and asked her if I could pray.

Many times being sensitive to the Holy Spirit can also come under the heading of the GIFT OF FAITH, but we share these stories with you to encourage you to listen for even the smallest little nudge from the Holy Spirit.

Several years ago we were in a western town and were standing by the book table, just casually talking to people and feeling the excitement of the meeting, when a young man came in carrying a boy who looked about nine or ten years old. He was also carrying a pair of small crutches. I asked the young man what the problem was with the boy. He said, "Ray has a spinal bifida, and I tried to get his parents to bring him, but they aren't believers, so I brought him myself." He went on to say, "He has never walked in his entire life, and I believe God is going to heal him!"

Something within my spirit leaped! I said, "Ray, there will be a time during the service tonight when I will call out your name. When I do, I want you to get up out of your seat and run to the front!" Speaking those words in the natural could be a problem, but the Holy Spirit had spoken to me, and I was just repeating what he had said!

I forgot all about Ray because he was sitting so far back I couldn't see him, when suddenly people started getting up out of wheel chairs. I turned and looked for Ray, but since I couldn't see him, I said, "Ray, wherever you are, get up right now in the name of Jesus and walk!"

Ray had been waiting all evening for that call! Hardly had the words come out of my mouth when Ray came out of what seemed like nowhere and came running up to the front! Being sensitive to the Holy Spirit, and being confident of the Holy Spirit can lead to exciting miracles!

A similar incident occurred in another city when I saw a beautiful black woman being pushed into a meeting in a wheel chair. A nudge (or shove) from the Holy Spirit prompted me to say to her, "During the service today I will read the 23rd Psalm. When I get to the part where it says, *'Yea, though I walk THROUGH the valley of the shadow of death, ...'* don't you dare SIT there. I want you to get up out of that wheel chair and run as fast as you can around this church!"

Little did I realize what the Holy Spirit had said! She never took her eyes off of me during the entire service, but sat in that wheel chair poised and ready to go! Toward the end of the service, I began to read the Psalm, and when I got to the part about walking THROUGH the valley, she didn't sit there, she leaped over the pedals of the wheel chair and began shouting at the top of her lungs as she ran around the church, out through the doors, into the narthex, and then down another aisle and up another one!

The only thing that finally stopped her running and shouting was when I met her in an aisle, touched her on the forehead, and she fell under the power of God, totally healed! She never went back in her wheel chair again! We saw her two years later, beautifully healthy because I had been sensitive to the Holy Spirit, and she had received the gift of faith!

You might think it isn't dignified to run around a church screaming. I don't either, but if you'd been stuck in a wheel chair for years, how would you react?

We were at a resort area one year and the last night of a crusade, faith was really spawned because of the miracles that had been happening all week, and the Holy Spirit very softly whispered, "Tell them that to-night everyone in a wheel chair is going to get out and walk!"

When I KNOW that I've heard from the Holy Spirit, I really get excited, so I shared with the audience in advance what was going to happen. When the Holy Spirit said, "Now!" I simply said, "I want everyone in wheel chairs to get up right now and walk to the front of the auditorium, in the name of Jesus!"

The next sixty seconds were probably the longest sixty seconds of my entire life, because not one person moved! Finally, after what seemed to me an hour, although it was probably no longer than the sixty seconds mentioned, the woman in the wheel chair closest to the front, got up and began to walk toward the stage. She had taken no more than two or three steps, when faith became alive in the person in the wheel chair behind her, and a man got up and began to walk!

One by one, one by one, every person in a wheel chair got up and walked that night! There were seven! Then a little girl came up wearing braces, and when Charles laid hands on her, the mother took the braces off, and the little girl began walking normally!

One of the things that is so exciting about being sensitive to the Holy Spirit is how it will start a flow of miracles! Hallelujah!

Be sensitive to God speaking to you. Listen to God's voice. It is far more important than anything you might learn about healing. Listen to God's voice. If he speaks to you, you will know that it is his voice, simply by the Spirit and by the Word of God. If you don't read the Word of God, you will not recognize God's voice and the devil will try to deceive you.

Don't be concerned about the devil if you are spending time in the Word of God. It is so very vital in healing the sick or operating in any of the gifts of the Spirit that you saturate your mind continually in the Word of God. Never let it get cold. Read it over and over, because every time you go back through the Bible, there is a freshness that comes and a new revelation of God's meaning.

Be sensitive to God. Learn to be acutely aware of the presence of God at all times so that you will be aware of the slightest little nudge from the Holy Spirit.

CHAPTER 15

CASTING OUT DEVILS

By Frances

Here is a subject which is extremely interesting, exciting, wild, stimulating, full of suspense and action, but is also an extremely dangerous one! Not dangerous to you as an individual, because you have more power than a demon, but dangerous because we can become overbalanced when we begin to deal in this area.

When I say, "Don't get overbalanced," I mean, don't say, "God has called me into a deliverance ministry!" We are called to be like Jesus. Jesus was a balanced individual. He spent PART of his time casting out demons; so you should spend PART of your time casting out demons, but not ALL of your time! Neither should you say, "Casting out demons is not MY ministry! Let someone else take care of that!" Because a portion of your ministry IS casting out demons, and you do not ever have to be afraid as long as you remember that the one who lives in you is greater than he that is in the world! You have power and authority over any demon you come up against. You always need to remember that!

Jesus cast out demons; Jesus healed the sick; Jesus taught; Jesus preached the gospel; Jesus studied the Word of God. Jesus did many things, so if you want to have a ministry that is balanced, and a ministry just like Jesus had, then you go and do likewise. You do ALL the things that Jesus did!

You might say, "I am a lady, and I am going to leave casting out demons to the men, because I do not want to wrestle with demons."

You do not have to wrestle with demons. Jesus simply said that those who believe shall use my authority — my name — to cast out demons. I cannot find anything in the Bible that says you have to wrestle all night with a demon. It merely says, *"In my name shall they cast out devils."* Matthew 8:16 says Jesus *"cast out the spirits with his word."* I believe he used only a few words at most to get them out. I believe what the scripture says, *"Greater is he that is in you, than he that is in the world"* (I John 4:4). I believe no demon in this world has as much power as I do. Do you know why I believe that? Because the Word says so, and that covers YOU as much as it does me!

Remember that each and every believer has been personally commissioned by the Lord Jesus Christ. To be a believer, you have to BELIEVE that you have the power within you to override anything the devil might throw at you.

Listen to what Jesus says in Luke 10:19, *"Behold, I give unto you power to tread on serpents and scorpions, and over all the power of the enemy: and nothing shall by any means hurt you."* The trouble with most of us is that we do not use the power that God has given us. The power is in us — we are endued with it, we are clothed with it, but we are afraid to reach up and touch it, or to step out and walk on spiritual water.

Don't be afraid to exercise the authority Jesus has given you! You will never cast out the first devil until you try. You might even be frightened the first time! I certainly was!

The first time I was ever called on to cast out a devil or run in the other direction, I stood my ground and cast out the devil. The man was an executive of one of the largest companies in America, and he lay on the floor writhing like a snake. The demon was trying to choke him, and after it came out, the man got up, looked at me and apologized. "I never knew that thing was in me," he said. He was a very well-educated and successful businessman, but a demon had control of his life!

Let me tell you what I did. I was shaking in my shoes, but while the man was on the floor, I just stood there and said, "Jesus, Jesus, Jesus!" I kept repeating the name over and over again simply because I didn't know what else to do! I had already commanded the spirit to come out. And that is all you really have to do, because Jesus said, *"IN MY NAME shall they cast out devils; they shall speak with new tongues; They shall take up serpents* (That does not mean going out in the bushes and picking up a rattlesnake, but if you do happen to find one, it means God would protect you if you were accidentally bitten by a snake); *and if they drink any deadly thing, it shall not hurt them* (If you were out on the mission field and someone slipped some poison in your water, you would not be harmed, but don't think you can deliberately pick up some strychnine and drink it and come out alive!); *they shall lay hands on the sick, and they shall recover."*

Jesus is not describing just a partial believer here. This isn't someone who thinks, "Healing passed away with the disciples." This is an all-the-way believer, someone who believes EVERYTHING the Bible says.

Let's look now at an incident in which Jesus cast out a devil: *"One of the men in the crowd spoke up and said, 'Teacher, I brought my son for you to heal — he can't talk because he is possessed by a demon. And whenever the demon is in control of him it dashes him to the ground and makes him foam at the mouth and grind his teeth and become rigid. So I begged your disciples to cast out the demon, but they couldn't do it.' Jesus said (to his disciples), 'Oh, what tiny faith you have, how much longer must I be with you until you believe? How much longer must I be patient with you? Bring the boy to me.' So they brought the boy, but when he saw Jesus the demon convulsed the child horribly, and he fell to the ground writhing and foaming at the mouth"* (Mark 9:17-20 TLB).

Many times when a demon-possessed person comes into the presence of a Holy Spirit-filled person, he will have a seizure, because that demonic spirit knows that he is going to have to go, and he's mad. That devil knows that he has come up against someone who has more power than he has; someone who knows his authority in Christ.

The devil knows whether YOU know that you have more power than he has. You can be a weak Christian and have the power of God in you, but if you do not believe that you have MORE power than he has, that devil is going to sit there and laugh in your face. He is going to say, "You have it, but you are so dumb that you do not know it. You just don't realize that you have that much power in you, so I am really smarter than you are!"

I have had many demons back up, and begin to say, "Don't touch me! I hate you! Don't come near me!" The person will usually put their arm across their face so as not to look at me, but do you know what I do? I go after the demon! Many times I have put my hand over a person's mouth and said, "In the name of Jesus, shut up!" And the demons have immediately shut up! Jesus said in Mark 1:25, *"Hold thy peace, and come out of him."* They often speak through a human voice, because they are then controlling the person's mind.

I don't have to listen to a demon, and neither do you. No demon is going to keep talking back to me, because I have more power than the demon has, and the demon knows that I know it! It takes authority to cast out a demon, and YOU HAVE TO KNOW THAT YOU HAVE THAT AUTHORITY!

Don't be surprised if you walk up to someone who has a demon in him, and the demon begins to scream and holler, because that's what some demons did when they saw Jesus. When you KNOW you are on the winning side, the devil is afraid of you.

When the spirit caused the child to fall to the ground, Mark tells us that Jesus asked the father, *"How long has he been this way?"*

"And he replied, 'Since he was very small, and the demon often makes him fall into the fire or into water to kill him. Oh, have mercy on us and do something if you can.' 'If I can?' Jesus asked. 'Anything is possible if you have faith.' The father instantly replied, 'I do have faith; oh, help me to have more.' When Jesus saw the crowd was growing he rebuked the demon. 'O demon of deafness and dumbness,' he said, 'I command you to come out of this child and enter him no more!' Then the demon screamed terribly and convulsed the boy again and left him; and the boy lay there limp and motionless, to all appearance dead. A murmur ran through the crowd — 'He is dead.' But Jesus took him by the hand and helped him to his feet and he stood up and was all right!" (Mark 9:21-27 TLB).

The demons at times tore the bodies or threw them to the ground before or as they came out. We have noticed that when we cast demons out, the person very frequently falls under the power of God, and because of the presence and power of the Holy Spirit, the demons depart. That is exactly what happened to the business executive in the story just related. JESUS WON THE BATTLE, AND SO CAN WE!

Matthew 28:18 says: *"And Jesus came and spake unto them, saying, 'ALL power is given unto me in heaven and in earth.'"*

God gave ALL power in HEAVEN and EARTH to Jesus, and then Jesus turned right around and said, "Now YOU go out and use my authority to cast out devils." That's right, he wants YOU to go, but I would suggest you never try it without the name and the authority of Jesus, and the baptism with the Holy Spirit, because I have news for you — you could really run into problems!

Let me share a very funny story about some people who were trying to do just that! Several years ago before we received the baptism, I went to a camp-meeting where I heard the wildest story I had ever heard. At that time I didn't even know that demons were real, so it was quite a shock to me when I heard that an old demon-possessed woman had been brought to the campmeeting for deliverance. A few men went into a building far away from the rest of the camp-meeting because this is where the deliverance was to take place. They were in there for just a short period of time when the noise and ruckus soon brought a lot of other men who got the surprise of their lives when they walked into the room!

Can you guess, using your wildest imagination, what she was doing? She was picking up strong, young men weighing from 150 to 200 pounds, and throwing them across the room! Do you know why she could do this? Because the men were in there without the power of the Holy Spirit. They were trying to use their own physical strength without the authority of Jesus! What happened? DISASTER, because I can assure you when you get a tiny, demon-possessed woman against people who do not have any power, what she can do to them is absolutely amazing!

Demons love to do that! They love to display their power, but they have to run when you use the name that is exalted above every other name! The name of Jesus is above demons! The name of Jesus is above cancer! The name of Jesus is above epilepsy. The name of Jesus is above every other name there is! That is a highly exalt-ed name!

The talk of this entire campmeeting was about this wild creature who had thrown big men around a room, and who had been sent home in the same condition in which she arrived, because none of them had the power that was greater than the one that was living in her!

I remember how frightened I was! I'm sure the story enlarged by the time it went around the campgrounds several times, but nevertheless, it was a real hair-curling story! How I wish I had known what I do today! I merely would have said, "Out in the name of Jesus," and the demon would have had to go.

This reminds me of one of the beautiful stories in the Bible which has a very funny twist concerning casting out demons without power. The nineteenth chapter of Acts tells us about the seven sons of Sceva who went about saying something like this: "We adjure you by Jesus whom Paul preaches to come out!"

The demon in the man who was possessed said, *"Jesus I know, and Paul I know, but who are you?"* He knew that Jesus and Paul had power and authority, but he knew these "Scevasons" didn't, so the demon just beat them to a pulp! They got the beating of their life! The demon was so powerful, he even ripped their clothes off!

That is almost the same thing that happened to the men who were trying to bring deliverance to this little old lady. They got their clothes torn and got the beating of their life! It might sound funny when we tell the story, but it certainly was not humorous to the men who were involved!

We learn by repetition! That is why we use Mark 16:17 over and over again because it is so vital that we remember this. I've discovered if you keep hearing the same thing over and over again, it eventually gets into your spirit; and suddenly you think, "Wow, I remember that now. That is a part of me!"

The great commission as related in Matthew is the

same as what Mark said, only Mark expanded it! *"Go ye into all the world, and preach the gospel to every creature. He that believeth and is baptized shall be saved; but he that believeth not shall be damned. And these signs shall follow them that believe; IN MY NAME SHALL THEY CAST OUT DEVILS; they shall speak with new tongues; They shall take up serpents; and if they drink any deadly thing, it shall not hurt them; they shall lay hands on the sick, and they shall recover"* (Mark 16:15-18).

In whose name do we cast out devils and heal the sick? In the name of Jesus! Remember that it is ALWAYS in the name of Jesus. We need to be aware of the fact that Jesus Christ lives in us by the power of the Holy Spirit. Jesus does not live out somewhere forty miles away. He does not drop by your house and drag you unwillingly down the road to eternal life or the fulfilling of the Great Commission! JESUS LIVES IN YOU! *"Christ IN you, the hope of glory"* (Col. 1:27).

Romans 8:11 says, *"But if the Spirit of him that raised up Jesus from the dead dwell IN you, he that raised up Christ from the dead shall also quicken your mortal bodies by his Spirit that dwelleth IN you."*

It is the positive, beyond-a-shadow-of-a-doubt knowledge that the Holy Spirit lives in us that is needed! The same resurrection power that brought Jesus out of the grave, is exactly the same power which indwells the Spirit-filled human! We need to get that fact into our spirits, and realize that we have exactly that same resurrection power! We don't have a lesser power, a lesser potency, but WE HAVE THAT SAME RESURRECTION POWER THAT BROUGHT JESUS RIGHT OUT OF THE GRAVE. I have it, and YOU have it if you have been baptized with the Holy Spirit. Let's act like it!

In acting on it, Matthew 12:28,29 is important to know in dealing with demons. Jesus said, *"But if I cast out devils by the Spirit of God, then the kingdom of God is come unto you. Or else how can one enter into a strong man's house, and spoil his goods, except he first bind the strong man? and then he will spoil his house."*

First, Satan needs to be bound in that powerful name of Jesus before you do anything else. When you do this, it is as though you cut the umbilical cord between Satan and his demons, and his little cohorts are left without the source of their power.

Satan is the prince of the air, and he is the commanding head of all fallen angels. Some people believe that demons and fallen angels are two separate kinds of beings. Truthfully, it does not make any difference whether you refer to them as demons, devils, fallen angels or evil spirits, they are all still under the control of Satan, because he is the ruler of the evil spirit world!

Once his power is bound in the name of Jesus, and his authority is superseded or controlled by the Spirit of God within us, then we can cast out the evil spirit, demon, or devil, whichever you prefer to call him, by the authority of Jesus!

Bringing this to a practical level, we believe incurable diseases are caused by a spirit in the majority of cases. When a doctor says there is no cure, our spiritual antennas pick up the fact that it is a spirit. For instance, because cancer is considered incurable, we believe it is caused by an evil spirit which attacks the body.

Let me show you how I understand the operation of a demon of cancer. He cannot get into your spirit if you are a Christian, but he can certainly come into and attack your body and your mind. A demon takes a look at a woman and says, "Wow, I think I will lay a little cancer on her. She looks like a real good victim." So he jumps into her body (not her spirit) and before long the woman discovers that she has cancer of the breast. She goes to the doctor. She panics!

The doctor says, "We will cut that cancer out." The demon goes right along into the operating room, and probably sits there laughing at the doctor, and watching him carefully. The minute the doctor inserts the knife, the demon says, "Whoops, here I go! I will go over to the other side." Then I imagine he just sits there and laughs as the doctor operates, because the damage of the demon has been done on one side.

He will gleefully say, "They think they have me, but they don't. I'll just jump over on the other side!"

Three years later the woman goes back, and they find cancer on the other side. Why? Because the demon has not been cast out, and you can't cut a demon out in surgery. When they do the next surgery, the demon says, "Whoops, I believe I will go into the stomach this time, or maybe I'll go into the lungs!"

Demons probably can plant a seed such as cancer into our flesh, bones or blood, and hover outside us, or even leave us, and the seed will continue to produce fast-growing, destructive cancer cells to destroy our bodies. When a male plants a sperm or seed into the womb of a female, cells develop into an infant. The devil counter-feits anything good with bad; therefore, it's logical that he would plant killer seeds instead of seeds of life. It is very likely that this is the way many diseases caused by demons are implanted into our bodies. We, of course, know from the Bible that demons do occupy human bodies when they can, so maybe they bring the seed and stay with it in the body.

We are told by doctors and nurses that the marrow of the bones is the manufacturer of blood, which is life. We know that cancer patients often need a new supply of blood.

Generally when we minister healing to a cancer victim, our prayers are something like, "Father, we praise you for the power you have given us over all the power of the enemy and for the power and authority to heal the sick. Satan, we bind you with the power of the Holy Spirit, in the name of Jesus. You spirit of cancer, we command you to come out and not return. We curse you, seed of cancer in this body, and command you to die. Marrow of the bones, we command you to produce healthy blood and send it forth for healing and health to this body. In the name of Jesus!"

A friend of ours who is a Spirit-filled surgeon has many patients referred to him because of his excellent record with cancer patients. When he gets in the operating room, he is the head "honcho" in there, so he lays hands on the patients and begins to pray in tongues before he operates, and then he casts out the spirit of cancer. He has a great recovery record, because once he commands and gets the spirit out, it is not hard to cut out the flesh that is diseased!

A friend of ours who is not only a successful medical doctor, but is Spirit-filled and ministers healing in the power of the Holy Spirit as well, was talking with us about incurable diseases being caused by evil spirits. He made this statement to us: "In this day and age in which we are landing men on the moon and are looking at DNA molecules through microscopes, I consider that those diseases which we cannot understand, and which we claim as incurable, must have their origin elsewhere than in science." (DNA molecules are chromosomes that carry the hereditary factors — genes — which are made of DNA.)

We believe that the "elsewhere than in science" is in the spirit world and the origin is demons.

"For we are not fighting against people made of flesh and blood, but against persons without bodies — the evil rulers of the unseen world, those mighty satanic beings and great evil princes of darkness who rule this world; and against huge numbers of wicked spirits in the spirit

world" (Eph. 6:12 TLB). We are not fighting against people! We are fighting against unseen powers. We cannot fight them in the natural as you would another human being.

When you are fighting against an evil spirit which causes a disease, you are fighting against an unseen principality. You are fighting against something you cannot see. That is why in the natural, we have absolutely no power or control over demons. Remember that it is only in the supernatural area where we win because of Jesus!

Remember that the attack from the devil comes in one of two places. It comes either into your body, or it comes into your mind. The devil wants your mind, and he will attack every way he can to try to get control of it. It is normally not your spirit that the devil attacks first, but if you let him get into your body, and you let him into your mind, then what do you think is going to happen to your spirit? Your spirit is going to go right down the drain with him! He wants your soul, but he attacks through your mind. The best defense is to start putting the Word of God into your mind so it will permeate your spirit. Then you can use the Word as a tool to fight off the attacks of the devil, and you can sit him down and say, "Look here, devil, IT IS WRITTEN ..."

There are many different kinds of spirits. Charles and I never mess around telling them to name themselves, because there was only one place in the Bible where Jesus ever asked them to name themselves, and they said, "Legion." Jesus did not continue by saying, "Legion, name yourself," because a legion could be a thousand or possibly thousands. Can you see Jesus sitting there listening to thousands of demons naming themselves? Jesus had more important things to do, and he used only a few words and they came out!

Our daughter Joan called home from college one time and said, "We had such an exciting Bible study tonight, and someone had the spirit of blab cast out!"

I said, "The spirit of what?"

She said, "The spirit of blab!"

Seems to me someone needed to be told to shut up and not talk so much! That also reminds me of the lady who wanted the spirit of "fat" cast out. The evangelist said, "This kind goeth not out but by prayer and fasting!"

Remember what I said about balance? We can get too extreme, and we can manufacture the names of all different kinds of spirits. I have heard about the spirits of sunburn, frostbite, cold and hot and many other interesting titles, but I do not believe these should be classed under the heading of evil spirits or demons!

Let us always remember, however, that there are many spirits that are legitimate. If you will notice, Jesus called spirits by what they did, not by names.

One of the spirits we have cast out successfully is a spirit of inheritance. At times, a curse will have been placed upon a family, and if you will trace their family history back far enough, you will find somewhere along the line they will say, "Oh, I remember my great grand-father had a curse placed on him," and that curse comes down to the present generation.

At a meeting on the west coast, there was a young man who was a member of a family of twenty-four children. FOURTEEN WERE DEAF! What does this say to you! This apparently came through a spirit of inheritance, because there would not have been the same set of circumstances surrounding each birth to make these children deaf. So there had to be something in the genes of the family. Who messes up the genes? The devil does!

This spirit of inheritance had come down through

this family, so we laid hands on him, bound Satan in the name of Jesus and by the power of God. After that, we cast out the spirit of inheritance and the deaf spirit. Then we asked God to create new ear drums. He must have had defective ear drums, or none at all, because for the first time in his life, the young man began to hear!

But with only ONE ear!

He came back the next day and reported what he had done the night before. He was so excited about hearing that he went into a restaurant where there were many people from the convention, and he went from table to table saying, "Say something, say something, I can hear!"

Then he got on the bus to go home and said to the driver, "I can hear!" Big deal! Well, maybe it would not be a big deal to you, because you have heard all of your life, but to someone who had never heard a sound, that was very exciting!

He had always hooked his alarm clock to his leg with an electric wire so it would shock him and wake him up, and the next day he said, "One of the most beautiful sounds I ever heard was the alarm going off!"

Notice how this was done. First of all, we bound Satan in the name of Jesus and by the power of God (See Matt. 12:29). We cast out the spirit of inheritance and deafness, and then we asked God for a creative miracle. James said, *"Ye ask, and receive not, because ye ask amiss"* (James 4:3), and many times people do not follow the ways of Jesus to heal the sick.

We could have prayed and commanded the spirit of inheritance to come out, and then forgotten to pray that the creative miracle would occur and he would be given a new ear. You would have gotten rid of the devil, but the man still might not have been able to hear because of the defect in the ears. Many miracles of healing occur instantly when the demon comes out. By the way, the second ear was healed the second night!

Please don't misunderstand what we say when we are talking about different ways to heal the sick, because GOD IS ALWAYS SOVEREIGN, and even if you prayed, "God heal his toe," and he didn't even have a toe, God could heal whatever was wrong with the person. Or even if there was nothing wrong with the toe, but the rest of the body had some defect in it, God could heal him, regardless of what you pray. Remember God is sovereign, and God can do exactly what he wants to do, but God wants US to do a lot more than we have been doing up until now!

At one of our services, our son-in-law Bob was called into an adjacent room where about fifty people were attempting to cast a demon out of a thirteen-year-old girl.

Some of the men were trying to hold this little girl on the floor, while others were loudly speaking in tongues and yelling, "Come out of her, you demon," and others were screaming, "Name yourself," over and over again.

There was so much confusion that the poor child would have been scared in the flesh until she wouldn't have known what to do if she had wanted to.

As a part of our team, Bob was asked to help, so he took charge and immediately asked everyone to leave the room except the little girl and her foster mother and father. Then Bob gently began to talk to the little girl to calm her.

Because of his experience in operating in the gifts of the Spirit, Bob knew that God could supply all his needs at a time like this, so he asked him for a word of knowledge about the spirit in the girl.

God spoke only one word — a surprising word — LAO.

Bob asked the girl what LAO meant to her.

She was astounded, and said, "How did you know about him?"

Bob said that God had told him.

Fearfully she said, "Nobody knows about him but me! He is the one who came to me and offered me the power and he is the one who tells me what to do. His name is LAO, and he tells me how to cause people to float up in the air and to make furniture and things float. He tells me how to do supernatural things in witchcraft." She said, "I'm scared!"

The little girl related that when she was only eight or nine years old a spirit offered her special powers if she would turn her life over to him. Just as Eve believed the lie of the devil, this girl believed a lie and made a deal with Satan. At first she thought it was "fun" to be able to operate in this power, but as time went on she became frightened.

Bob asked her if she would like to be free of this devil control of her life. She said, "Do you really mean I could be free without him destroying me with the same powers he has given to me?" Bob assured her that if she really wanted freedom, he could bind the spirit so that it could not use its powers over her. He told her that Jesus said in Luke 10:19, *"Behold, I give unto you power to tread on serpents and scorpions, and over all the power of the enemy: and nothing shall by any means hurt you."*

She said, "I want to be set free."

Bob very softly, but with belief and authority, commanded the spirit to come out in the name of Jesus! And the spirit came out and she was completely set free from this tormenting demon.

We saw her about a year later and she was a beautiful Christian, happy, and with no fear in her life!

Glory to God, he set her free!

Through this word from God, the confidence of the little girl was won and she was willing to talk freely to Bob.

What would have happened if Bob had commanded

the spirit in her to name itself? The Bible gives that answer: *"Ye are of your father the devil, and the lusts of your father ye will do. He was a murderer from the beginning, and abode not in the truth, because there is no truth in him. When he speaketh a lie, he speaketh of his own: for he is a liar, and the father of it"* (John 8:44).

If the devil cannot tell the truth, how can we ask him or one of his demons to name itself and expect the truth? Isn't it more scriptural to ask God?

"Our words are wise because they are from God ... But we know about these things because God has sent his Spirit to tell us, and his Spirit searches out and shows us all of God's deepest secrets" (I Cor. 2:7, 10 TLB).

Please don't feel that we are criticizing those who successfully exorcise demons by other ways than we use. If you have succcess making demons name themselves, keep on doing it! But do try an easier way occasionally, will you?

If you have success wrestling with a demon all night long, I suppose it's all right to continue, but I'd certainly find a short cut so I could spend more time talking about Jesus rather than demons.

I believe God is in heaven crying over churches where they do not lay hands on people on Sunday morning and believe for their healing, because God wants you well!

We were at Bob Tilton's Word of Faith World Outreach Center in Dallas, Texas, on a Christmas Sunday. The people were giving testimonies, but it seemed to me that almost everyone gave a testimony about prosperity! Finally, at the end, one lady got up and said, "I was healed of cancer this year."

After the service I said to Bob, "Don't very many people get healed in your church?"

He said, "Not many."

I said, "How come?"

He said, "I teach them how to walk in divine health so they don't need to get healed."

Glory to God! I think that is how we should be in churches. We ought to walk in divine health so we don't have to be healed, but we are teaching you these different ways to heal the sick so you can go around the world, or in your part of the world, where the people don't know how to walk in divine health, and heal them! They may have never even heard that there is healing in the name of Jesus! When God said, *"Beloved, I wish above all things that thou mayest prosper and be in health, even as thy soul prospereth"* (III John 2), he meant he wanted us to walk in divine health!

God will often do the unusual when you first receive the baptism or when you first start to go out and lay hands on the sick. Did you know that? God probably says, "Well, I am going to see if they really mean business with me."

In our hometown area, shortly after we received the baptism, Charles and I were speaking in a little church, and a man brought a lady who had cancer. Remember, we had just received the baptism, and we had not been raised in Pentecost.

We did not understand the supernatural!

We did not understand falling under the power! These were new things to us, and yet it was so exciting to suddenly realize that when you put out your hand, someone fell over! To walk down the aisle of a church and see people fall over under the power of God was a tremendously thrilling and awesome experience!

We were so excited because of the things we had begun to see Jesus do, that nothing could hold us back! Charles and I laid hands on this sick woman and prayed for her, and she went under the power of God! We said, "Thank you, Jesus," and she began to throw up! It did not seem to bother her in the least. NOR DID IT

BOTHER US, because something in our spirits said, "That which is coming out is the cancer!"

About two bucketsful came out, and all the time we were standing there saying, "Hallelujah! Glory to God!" If you don't think it will test your faith to see a whole mound of horrible looking stuff come out, you had better think again! God wanted to show us that he does things whatever way he wants to whether you think you are too lady-like or not to stand there and see someone vomit!

It was the most awful-looking mess I ever saw, but glory to God, the cancer came OUT of her instead of staying IN her!

God doesn't always do things like that, but in the beginning he can certainly test your faith! He said, "Are you sure you want to be in the healing ministry? Are you sure this is what you want?" Charles and I said, "Yes," and we kept right on!

The same thing happened in a huge modernistic church after one great service we held there one night when more than seven hundred people were healed at one time. One man who had just been Spirit-filled came up to us and said, "How do I explain to the janitors who don't know anything about the healing power of God, why all that cancer was vomited all over the floor last night!"

I have heard that at some of Aimee Semple McPherson's meetings they had to come in with a wheelbarrow and shovel up the cancers that fell off people. Don't turn up your nose at it! Just wait until you are there and some cancer lump falls off in your hands! Do you know what will happen to you? The Spirit of God will overcome you at that time, and you will look at that nasty cancer and say, "Hallelujah!" Because it is dead and just lying in your hands! It is not living on the body of someone else!

Would you like to lay hands on someone and have

the cancer come off in your hands? I tell you, that is real living! You might think that going out to dinner at a real fancy place, and having all kinds of steak and lobster to eat is really living, but that is not what living is all about. Real living is seeing the sick healed and the demons flee even if their evidence ends up in your hands! We rarely see people vomit when they are healed and delivered, but don't be shocked if this does happen!

When Jesus arose from the dead, he left an eternally defeated Satan behind him. Never think of Satan as anything except a defeated foe. Don't get out there and think, "Greater is he that is looking at me through the eyes of that girl who has a demon in her than he that is in me. I think I had better back off. I think I had better run someplace else." Don't you dare ever think like that. Remember the devil is an eternally defeated foe!

Again, I want to issue a warning. The deliverance ministry is exciting because of the tremendous freedom it brings to people. But don't ever get so lopsided that you see a demon on every door knob. We have new carpet in the City of Light, and it is "fuzzing" all over the place. Now that is not a demon of "carpet fuzz" because it is just something that happens when you get a new carpet, and you don't vacuum it every day! Do you see what I'm saying? There is a real valid place, and a real valid time, and a real valid demonic spirit for you to cast out. And there is a sufficient number of real live evil spirits around so you don't have to run around trying to make up demons of all kinds!

Here's a little warning that might help you. From time to time, a mother will bring her child to me and say something like this: "This child is possessed of demons. I can't do anything with him. He needs deliverance!"

She is holding a screaming, kicking, scratching child, and he is so wild I can't even get close to him.

One day God showed me why some of these children react like this. How would you like to have some powerful evangelist lay hands on you for something you didn't understand, shake you all over the place and command, "Devil, you come out of him!" It would frighten you so much, you would probably decide right on the spot that you would never let anyone else pray for you the rest of your life!

We saw an example of this recently when a mother of a boy about nine or ten tried to present him to me bodily. She said, "He's got 47 demons left in him. Get them out of him!"

I looked at the child, and he only appeared frightened to me, but when the child looked at me, he broke loose from his mother and ran completely around a huge auditorium so fast that nobody could catch him. He was screaming at the top of his lungs, and yet I couldn't see anything but a normal child who was frightened.

That's when God spoke and told me that this child had not been prepared for a healing touch of God, the loving Father. God asked me how I'd like it if someone dropped me on the floor and had ten adults sit down on top of me to hold me down? You'd better believe I'd begin fighting and scratching and kicking and doing everything else I could think of to get free, and I'm not demon possessed at all.

A man saw the same thing I did, and the next day he sat down with this same child and with great love prayed that the scars of careless deliverance would be erased from his mind. This particular child was beautifully set free through love, not deliverance.

By Charles

As Frances and I write this book, we are constantly keeping in our minds that the ways of God are past finding out, and that his wisdom and power are beyond any possible way of expressing, and that we have caught only a glimpse of how he does things. We can't even begin to comprehend things God takes for granted — like creating a universe, and placing stars and planets into an exact orbit.

We are simply describing and sharing with you ways that God has worked and is working in our ministry, many of which are strikingly similar to ways he worked in episodes recorded in his Word.

We are describing ways and examples of casting out demons. There are no doubt hundreds of ways you can go about it, but we know it finally boils down to the principle that it is done by the power of God's Holy Spirit in us, and that it is done in the name of Jesus, and that it is done by the authority of Jesus! Everything else we describe is to encourage you and to teach you ways of going about performing the commission of Jesus to free the oppressed so that they can be brought into the kingdom of light.

A lady who had pain in her abdomen for three years had been to many kinds of doctors and none of them could find any cause for the pain. She had been prayed for in many charismatic meetings, and still the pain persisted. We praise God for our medical profession, but I reasoned that if the doctors could not find the cause, it must be a demon, because doctors without the baptism with the Holy Spirit do not have the supernatural discernment to know that a spirit can cause pain.

I asked her to place her hands where the pain was,

and I laid my hand on top of hers, bound Satan, and commanded the spirit of pain to come out in the name of Jesus.

I saw her released from pain, and so I asked her what happened. God must have opened her spirit eyes, because when I said "Out" she replied, "What appeared to be a large thing like a leech with legs dug into me came out, turned over in the air and zoomed out into space away from me." All pain instantly left! Praise Jesus for freeing the captives!

A few months later we were visited by a friend who said his wife had a pain in her abdomen, that she had been to many different kinds of doctors and they could find no cause or cure, and that she had been prayed for many times. The situation was exactly like the other lady.

They lived about 400 miles away, so I asked him to call his wife on the phone. I explained to her about the other deliverance. She placed her hand on the pain area, I bound Satan by the power of the Holy Spirit, and commanded the spirit of pain to come out, in Jesus' name. When I asked, "Where is the pain?" she replied, "I DON'T HAVE IT ANY MORE!"

Glory to God, even distance doesn't make any difference when the authority of Jesus is used to rid someone of an enemy of God!

By the way, both of those from whom a spirit of pain was cast out were Spirit-filled Christians. It is possible that the deaf, dumb, blind, or other spirits Jesus named could have been cast out of a believer. Again, we do not believe a demon can be in the spirit of a Christian, but that they can attack a body or mind. We know of no evidence that the demon actually has to "dwell in" a person to cause a "spirit of pain" or any of the other spirits Jesus named. They can simply attack a part of the body, possibly even to implant cancer into the body.

I was talking with a man one day who told me that his right leg had been amputated above the knee. That night he came to me for prayer, and said he had pain in his right foot.

I started to lay hands on him when I suddenly remembered that he was the one with no right leg or foot. I said, "What do you mean, pain in your right foot — I thought you told me you didn't have one?"

He said, "That's right. The doctors call this a phantom pain."

The thought immediately came into my mind that there were no human nerves left to signal pain to the brain, so it had to be a phantom spirit. I commanded that phantom spirit of pain to come out in the name of Jesus and by the power of the Holy Spirit, and IT INSTANTLY LEFT!

Then God gave me a word of knowledge that the pain would return twice more, and that he was to rebuke it each time, and after that he would never have it again.

The next day he came to me to say, "You were exactly right; it came back twice; each time I rebuked it and it left!"

Is all pain caused by a demon? No, because if you stick your finger on a hot stove or cut it with a knife, it will pain you. If this occurs, command it to be healed in the name of Jesus, and rebuke the pain.

When Jesus went to Peter's mother-in-law's house, she was sick of a fever. Jesus took her by the hand (touched her) and in Luke it is recorded that he stood over her, and rebuked the fever; and it left her (Luke 4:39).

Our daughter, Joan, had two wisdom teeth pulled when she was a teenage girl. By the time I came home from work, the effect of the Novocain had worn off, and Joan was crying with pain. I put my hands on her jaws and said, "Pain, I rebuke you in the name of Jesus." The pain left and never returned. This was not a spirit, just an injury through surgery.

We have ministered in audiences across the world, and when the power of God is flowing and the people are responsive to the sharing of the Word of God and to the testimonies of his great miracles, demons simply cannot stand his presence. They just leave their human habitations.

One night in a large crowd, people were falling under the power by the scores, they were getting healed in masses, the gift of the word of knowledge was working through us, and a hideous scream came forth from the back of the audience.

Someone had brought an unsaved friend from a dance studio, and the demon could not stand the power of God, so it left without being told to do so.

It is very important that all of us do everything we can to win those ensnared by the thief and the destroyer before they are destined to be forever lost from the glory God has provided for us.

Oh, if we could all get a vision of what God wants for us, and realize the marvel of it all when we fully realize that we are a chosen generation, a special people who are called by God. He doesn't want us bound by the devil, he wants us set free by his holy and awesome power!

"Thus saith the Lord God of Israel, Let my people go ..." (Ex. 5:1). God was delivering his people from a devil-controlled Pharaoh. And God wants us to deliver his people from a devil-controlled world.

One of the most beautiful deliverances I have ever seen happened in our office. A young lady was brought to me who had repeatedly attempted suicide. She was determined to kill herself. She was totally possessed by this controlling demon of suicide. She had been counseled by Spirit-filled Christians; she had gone through inner healing; she had been prayed for, and attempts had been made to cast the demon out, but she was still determined to kill herself.

She had a bitterness toward life so strong that her determined desire for destruction plainly showed up in her face!

She had been confined to a psychiatric ward of the hospital, and even there attempted suicide, and had even committed adultery in the hospital.

As I began to minister to her with a God-given love and compassion, I very softly told her that God loved her and wanted her to live for him and be in heaven with him for eternity. I told her that the devil was the one who was causing her to feel so defeated and depressed, and that God could bring peace and happiness to her even here on earth. I explained that heaven was wonderful and beautiful, and then described how hell is horrible and tormenting — even much worse than the "hell" she was living in now.

Then I told her that if she would just ask Jesus to forgive her, he would erase and remove all of this from her.

She whiningly said, "I'm so confused that I don't know what to do."

I explained to her that she was not the one telling me that she was confused; that this was an evil spirit in her that was using her mind and her voice.

Again, speaking very softly, I explained that the devil wanted her to commit suicide so that the murder of herself would take her into his eternal control in hell, and she would have no further opportunity to be freed from the devil's control.

Again I invited her to make the simple choice of going to the tormenting hell, or of having eternal peace and joy in heaven.

Again she whimpered and said, "I just can't think."

She was sitting in a chair and I was standing in front of her. I gently put my fingers under her chin and lifted her head so I could look into her eyes.

The Spirit of God had anointed me with a supernatural love and desire to win her soul from the demon who was trying to rob her from God with this last desperate attempt.

I said, "I'm going to command the spirit that is talking to me out of your mouth to come out, and IT WILL COME OUT, and then you can think straight to make your choice for Jesus."

In almost a whisper, but with power and authority, I said, "Devil, I bind you in the name of Jesus and by the power of the Holy Spirit, and command you, you spirit of suicide and you spirit of bitterness, come out of her!"

There was no yelling, no loud voice, no fighting, no struggle, no vomiting, no resistance, no evidence of seeing anything come out; but in a soft, believing, knowing voice, the command which Jesus told us to use was given, and the young lady's whole countenance changed in an instant. A peace came on her face, a softness in her eyes, and a transformation came upon her so mighty that she hardly looked like the same bitter, devil-controlled woman who sat there a moment before.

Then I simply, softly said to her, "Say, Jesus, forgive my sins!" She repeated those ever-so-powerful words from her heart with "her" voice which was now controlled by her mind instead of by the demon. "Jesus, come into my heart and make me the kind of woman you want me to be. Be my Savior; be my Lord. I love you Father; I love you Jesus!"

She left the office a few minutes later, loving Jesus, loving God as her spiritual Father, and with a Bible and some of our books in her hand.

"And they come to Jesus, and see him that was possessed with the devil, and had the legion, sitting, and clothed, and in his right mind: and they were afraid" (Mark 5:15).

THANK YOU, JESUS!

Depression or oppression is a state of the mind, but can be influenced by a demon. Demons can deal with the thoughts of mankind, and consequently have an ability to cause you to think unclean thoughts. Therefore, they must also be able to attack the mind with thoughts causing depression or oppression, generally arising from some selfish attitude.

"If you are angry, don't sin by nursing your grudge. Don't let the sun go down with you still angry — get over it quickly; for when you are angry you give a mighty foothold to the devil" (Eph. 4:26 TLB). The Bible tells us to get over anger — that means we can do it if we are willing. If we are not willing, it gives a foothold to demonic activity and could lead to possession by the demon through total control of our mind and eventually our spirit and soul. Then there can be no dwelling of Christ within us.

The demoniac who had the legion cast out, was back in his right mind afterwards. This indicates that the possessed man had his mind controlled by the demon (Mark 5:15).

What causes people to follow Satan and his evil ways? How do people submit themselves to a hating devil when God has so much for us? Why would anyone even consider making a deliberate choice to submit themselves to an eternity of torment instead of an eternal home with God?

"The thief cometh not, but for to steal, and to kill, and to destroy: I am come that they might have life, and that they might have it more abundantly" (John 10:10).

The trickery of Satan is to pervert our minds into believing that his way is best. If we accept his lies, it is the beginning of the invitation by mankind for a demon to kill and destroy their souls by stealing them away from God. He does this principally through bad attitudes, and BAD ATTITUDES ARE NOT DEMONS, but they give a foothold to demonic activity. Bad attitudes don't need to be cast out like a spirit, but we need to overcome them by the power of God!

The devil lied to Eve in the Garden of Eden, and she had the choice of rejecting his temptation, or believing his lie. She gave a foothold to the devil, and he stole her away from God. Satan cleverly gained this foothold through her mind. He cunningly put thoughts or words into her mind and she believed him.

When you are ministering to someone in the deliverance of demons, first talk with them to see if they are saved. Ask them if they really love Jesus and if they would say, "Jesus is Lord of my life." If they are truly born again, they will be able to say that and mean it, but if they are not able to say it, you need to deal with a demon. Otherwise, inquire about attitudes that are wrong. MAYBE THEY JUST NEED TEACHING about their responsibility to get rid of bad attitudes. *"Here is the test: no one speaking by the power of the Spirit of God can curse Jesus, and no one can say, 'Jesus is Lord,' and really mean it, unless the Holy Spirit is helping him"* (I Cor. 12:3 TLB).

A woman came to Frances one night with a very sad story. She started off by saying, "I've been prayed for by the best, so I don't know why I'm coming to you, but ...

I've had the demon of smoke cast out!

I've had the demon of tobacco cast out!

I've had the demon of nicotine cast out!

I've had the demon of cigarettes cast out!" She continued, "Do you have a word from the Lord for me?"

Frances said, "Yes!"

"What is it?" she asked.

Frances said, "Quit!"

The woman was obviously shocked. But too many times we blame spirits or demons for things that are simply our fault. We run from evangelist to evangelist, from preacher to preacher, from conference to conference, asking for deliverance at every service, when the problem is really very simple. It lies within ourself — QUIT SINNING! Throw those cigarettes away, don't buy any more, and quit blaming it on demons!

If, with all your heart, mind, body and soul, you want to be obedient to all that God and Jesus want you to do, there will never be a desire to sin. A desire to sin is simply a way of expressing your disbelief that God's way is best. God doesn't like that. But it delights him when you want to do what pleases him!

"I advise you to obey only the Holy Spirit's instructions. He will tell you where to go and what to do, and then you won't always be doing the wrong things your evil nature wants you to. For we naturally love to do evil things that are just the opposite from the things that the Holy Spirit tells us to do; and the good things we want to do when the Spirit has his way with us are just the opposite of our natural desires. These two forces within us are constantly fighting each other to win control over us, and our wishes are never free from their pressures."

"When you are guided by the Holy Spirit you need no longer force yourself to obey Jewish laws."

"But when you follow your own wrong inclinations your lives will produce these evil results: impure thoughts, eagerness for lustful pleasure, idolatry, spiritism (that is, encouraging the activity of demons), hatred and fighting, jealousy and anger, constant effort to get the best for yourself, complaints and criticisms, the feeling that everyone else is wrong except those in your own little group — and there will be wrong doctrine, envy, murder, drunkenness, wild parties, and all that sort of thing. Let

me tell you again as I have before, that anyone living that sort of life will not inherit the kingdom of God" (Gal. 5:16-21 TLB).

Do you notice from that part of God's Word that these are attitudes which come into our mind because our old self-nature wants its way? That is the simplest way I know to tell you how the devil gets a foothold on your mind in his drive to take your soul away from God.

The way to avoid the trap the devil sets is simply set forth in the rest of that chapter: *"But when the Holy Spirit controls our lives he will produce this kind of fruit in us: love, joy, peace, patience, kindness, goodness, faithfulness, gentleness and self-control; and here there is no conflict with Jewish laws. Those who belong to Christ have nailed their natural evil desires to his cross and crucified them there. If we are living now by the Holy Spirit's power, let us follow the Holy Spirit's leading in every part of our lives. Then we won't need to look for honors and popularity, which lead to jealousy and hard feelings"* (Gal. 5:22-26 TLB).

When we let thoughts contrary to God's nature enter into our minds, these thoughts begin to develop and become a part of us. Our inner desires either invite the Holy Spirit or Satan's old nature in us to control our thoughts.

Stop thinking about the negative, evil old nature and you can stop most demons from having activity in your mind. They don't immediately possess you, but they begin to control you little by little until you no longer desire God's ways.

"Submit yourselves therefore to God. Resist the devil, and he will flee from you. Draw nigh to God, and he will draw nigh to you. Cleanse your hands, ye sinners; and purify your hearts, ye double minded" (James 4:7,8). Who is to do that? We are.

One day before Frances and I were married, I was

driving from one part of Houston to another while I was working as a Certified Public Accountant. The sun was shining, I was happy, I was singing songs of praise to God, and the whole world was thrilling to live in. I stopped in the bright sunlight at a parking lot, got out of the car and started toward a cafeteria for lunch.

My life had been totally surrendered to God and I had spent over a thousand exciting hours meditating in the Bible the past few months. Everything was beautiful and perfect!

But as I stepped out of the car, a darkness, a depression came over me and it felt like everything was wrong, that all love left me, all joy and peace left, and that my whole world had caved in on me.

I didn't know what had happened. It was so sudden and my mind tried in a flash of a second to know what had happened.

But, because my mind had been saturated with the Word of God, and was controlled by the Holy Spirit, and my desires were to please God and not myself, a scripture came quickly into my mind.

I said, "God, if that is the devil, get him out of here and draw close to me!"

Instantly, like a flash of lightning, all the darkness, the depression, the emptiness left me like a wind. The evil spirit which had so viciously attacked my mind could actually be sensed like a wind which for an instant rose out of me slowly and then it accelerated to a tremendous speed and disappeared into space.

Satan had sent a demon after me to try to get into my spirit to control me and to steal me away from the God I loved so much.

But, *"the word of God is quick, and powerful, and sharper than any twoedged sword, piercing even to the dividing asunder of soul and spirit, and of the joints and marrow, and is a discerner of the thoughts and intents of the heart"* (Heb. 4:12).

The great weapon against demons is the Word of God. That is one reason we should meditate day and night in his Word, and think about him and what will please him; not think about what we can get for ourselves.

"For though we walk in the flesh, we do not war after the flesh: (For the weapons of our warfare are not carnal, but mighty through God to the pulling down of strong holds;) Casting down imaginations, and every high thing that exalteth itself against the knowledge of God, and bringing into captivity every thought to the obedience of Christ" (II Cor. 10:3-5).

The first time a demon attacks your thoughts is the time to get rid of it! Don't let it get a foothold on your mind or your thoughts. Preventive medicine is better than having to take medication for a cure. The Word of God is the immunization we need to protect us from demonic influence, control or possession. We need to have the nature of God implanted in us as an inoculation against the infection the devil places in our thoughts and inner desires.

Demons are invisible, bodiless creatures that have the ability to move about wherever Satan sends them, and they can hover over us, surround us, attack us, put thoughts into our minds, put diseases into our bodies, or even cause us to lose our minds and become insane.

They can be present at our birth, or as we are formed in the belly of our mothers, and cause defects in our formation. Being spirits who live forever, they can transfer from one generation to another and thus cause diseases or defects which may be in the form of genes or deformations.

They come against our flesh to try to control our souls. We must use all the understanding we can get, and allow the Holy Spirit to teach us how to get rid of them, in whatever way they attack.

Your job and our job is to liberate our fellow human

beings from the influence and control of Satan and his demon aides, and to teach them how to remain FREE!

"Heal the sick, cleanse the lepers, raise the dead, CAST OUT DEVILS: freely ye have received, freely give" (Matt. 10:8).

I believe that God is preparing a body of people to go out in mighty power. Why? His heart is crying out because he knows that people need to be healed and delivered!

God is saying to his people, "I want a bunch of believers who are willing to go out and know they are not wrestling against human beings, but against principalities and powers. They are going to go out in the name of Jesus and lay hands on the sick with results for me! And they are going to be victorious!"

Do you know there are people crying all over the world, "Somebody teach me the gospel. Somebody teach me how you can get healed." That is why it is so easy to heal the sick when you go overseas. Glory to God, they just come believing!

And they do love to heal the sick! A friend of ours just returned from Haiti where he said many of the pastors do not even own a Bible, because they do not know how to read, but you give them a scripture like, *"They shall lay hands on the sick, and they shall recover"* or *"And these signs shall follow them that believe; In my name shall they cast out devils"* and they go on the run! They take a scripture like one of those, lay hands on the sick and tremendous healings take place! Once they hear the Word, they get it into their spirits and never try to disprove it, they only try to act upon it!

I can hardly wait until readers put these principles into practice, and letters start coming back here saying, "I went here and I went there, and I was in this foreign country, and I was in that foreign country, and people got healed all over the place!"

You might think that is not a reality, but with my heart and soul I believe it is! I believe God is going to take people who ACT, to places they never dreamed of in their entire life, and begin using them to heal the sick! THIS MEANS YOU!

CHAPTER 16

THE GIFT OF FAITH

By Frances

One morning as we were preparing to teach on different ways to heal the sick, the Lord spoke to me and said something which I believe can divinely change your life and your ministry where healing is concerned.

Can each and every one of us have the power to heal the sick? Yes, the Word says that the ability to heal is within each and every believer! (Mark 16:18).

But you may say, "I don't have the gift of healing, because it hasn't been given to me by the Holy Spirit, and he gives the gifts as he wills!"

God spoke to me and said, "The Holy Spirit gives gifts as he wills, and HE GIVES THEM TO 'WHO-SOEVER WILL!'"

He is not going to give you a gift if you're not going to use it!

He is not going to let the gift of faith drop down on you if you are going to be a spiritual chicken and not do what he tells you to do.

He is not going to give you the gift of faith to tell someone to rise up out of a wheel chair, if your answer is going to be, "God, you've got to be kidding, because I might be embarrassed if it didn't work!"

The gift of faith is one of the exciting gifts present-ed to us by the Holy Spirit. It is not a gift that is present at all times, but a gift that makes you rise over supernatural barriers without any doubt and perform a miracle! The gift of faith will make you such a mighty person of valour that you can hardly believe when it's all over that you were the one who did it!

The gift of faith transforms you for a period of time into a supernatural person. The exciting story in the third chapter of Acts points this out when Peter said, *"Silver and gold have I none; but such as I have give I thee: In the name of Jesus Christ of Nazareth rise up and walk!"* The gift of faith had fallen on Peter, and he became a supernatural person, for the Word says, *"And he took him by the right hand and lifted him up: and immediately his feet and ancle bones received strength."* The gift of faith was poured out upon Peter, and ALSO ACTED UPON BY HIM, because he was one of those who "will!"

The gift of faith is something you will immediately sense when it falls! For one brief moment, the devil will take his last fling and there may be a flicker of doubt in your mind, but step out in faith, and become a supernatural person!

We were not raised in Pentecost, so until we received the baptism with the Holy Spirit, we had seen only a few healings. After the baptism, healings began to increase until God suddenly dropped us into the miracle ministry in El Paso, Texas, and as a result we wrote the book, SINCE JESUS PASSED BY. One day in Louisville, Kentucky, a Catholic couple was reading this book. They could hardly believe that God was still doing supernatural things today. But they had a little boy who had cerebral palsy. He had never walked without braces and crutches in his entire life. He had never crawled, because he had no motor coordination. The more they read, the more faith began to rise up in them! Could their five-year-old be healed in the 20th century?

They remembered they had seen an ad in a newspaper that we were having a miracle service in Louisville at Evangel Tabernacle. Excitement filled the air as they made plans to come. They lived on a farm, so they got up at 3 AM and milked their cows. Everyone dressed in a hurry, got into the car and drove about one hundred and twenty slow-moving miles to get to the church by 8 AM because they didn't want to miss the miracle service, regardless of what time it was to start.

All they talked about on the way to Louisville was Jeffie's healing! Never a negative statement! All positive talk! JEFFIE WAS GOING TO BE HEALED!

They were disappointed when they got there because they discovered the miracle service was scheduled for that night, and they couldn't stay because the cows had to be milked again; however, we promised them that we would pray for Jeffie sometime during the morning service.

We looked at that crippled little body, and our faith wasn't very high. It was a small morning crowd without great numbers of believers to help build our faith, when suddenly the healing power of God began to flow like a river, and God dropped the supernatural gift of faith down on both of us, on Jeffie's parents, and also on a little five-year-old boy.

I ran into the audience, picked Jeffie up, and told his parents to come forward. I held Jeffie on my lap, and asked him an important question, "Do you believe God can heal you?"

Jeffie looked at me like I had lost my mind, because all the way to Louisville his parents had been telling him he was going to be healed, and here I was asking him if he thought that God could heal him!

He said, "Oh, yes, he's going to heal me today!" No hesitation, no doubt, no questioning, no nothing, just absolute faith without a doubt!

The gift of faith was churning up in us. We laid hands on Jeffie, and then Charles turned to his parents and asked them if they would like to take his braces off, and just as soon as they said "Yes," they both fell under the power, so Charles removed Jeffie's braces.

He took Jeffie off of my lap, held him in a standing position, and with no hesitation at all said, "Jeffie, in the name of Jesus, RUN!"

He didn't tell him to walk; he told him to run! And there were three steps down from the platform to the floor.

Jeffie never hesitated.

He leaped down the three steps and began to run!

He never doubted that he could run!

He never doubted that he was healed!

He just ran as fast as he could! Not too well for the first 20 to 30 feet, but gradually increasing in speed and ability! For those first few steps, his hips were crooked, and his gait unsteady, but before long he reached the back and turned around. I said, "Run back here Jeffie!" and he took off and ran for the pulpit as fast as he could. I stepped down to the floor level with my arms outstretched, and when he was about six feet away, he made a flying leap, climbed right up me like I was a ladder, and wrapped his little legs around my waistline!

This was the crippled child who had never walked without braces in his entire life!

THE GIFT OF FAITH was not only given, but received by ALL!

We ate lunch with Jeffie and his parents and they gave us his braces because they knew he would never need them again. They still sit in the foyer of our home as a beautiful, modern testimony of the power of God! He went shopping in his stocking feet and got his first pair of Hush Puppies, something he had wanted all his life!

When we were with Jeffie a year later, he had gained twenty-five pounds. In one year his shoe size had gone from a children's size eleven to a "man's" size three, and he made the honor roll in school.

God had healed him completely, mind, body and spirit!

What would have happened if we hadn't exercised the gift of faith?

I believe that Jeffie would never have been healed!

I believe that if Charles had sat back and said, "I can't ask that child to walk because he's never walked without braces," that Jeffie would still be in braces today.

The gift of faith is something that just wells up and wells up within you, and whenever it does, step out like a wild tiger, and do whatever God says to do. Some of our greatest healings have come through the gift of faith, and the same things can happen to you!

We were in Calloway Gardens, Georgia, at a convention of the Full Gospel Business Men. As we entered the room, Dr. Doug Fowler, a surgeon from Jacksonville, Florida, was giving a prophecy that ended something like this, "Tonight I am going to do creative miracles! I am going to put parts in bodies that are not there! Thus saith the Lord!"

Hallelujah, did we ever get excited! We probably got more than naturally or normally excited because it was such an unusual prophecy to come out of a medical doctor who knows what it takes for a creative miracle, because doctors know that creative miracles don't happen on operating tables where they take things out, but where it is hard to get something back in that isn't there.

The first thing we did that night was to grow out short arms to demonstrate the Spirit and power (I Cor. 2:4). The ushers brought up a man who had one arm that was probably eight or nine inches shorter than the other one. We asked him what caused this, and he said, "When I was about twelve years old, my arm was almost severed at the shoulder, and they sewed it back on. It lived, but it never grew after that!"

Both of us felt something explode within us! We had both heard the prophecy about new parts, and we both wanted to minister to the man instantly, because BOTH OF US RECEIVED THE GIFT OF FAITH simultaneously! When two people receive it, that is something electrifying!

There he stood with one forty-year-old arm, and one twelve-year-old arm. Charles held the two arms out, and with three medical doctors standing behind us, Charles commanded the muscle, tissue, veins, marrow, ligaments, skin, bone and other parts to be put in, and in front of some thirteen hundred people he commanded that arm to GROW, GROW, GROW!

There was no doubt or unbelief in either of us! The arm responded to the command given through the gift of faith, and it began to grow, grow, GROW!

Those three medical doctors began to cry unrestrainedly because they knew what an impossibility it was to see what they were actually seeing! In approximately fifteen seconds, God had put new parts into that arm. GOD DID IT AGAIN!

What happened as a result?

A woman got so excited, that she came right out of her wheel chair! She forgot she couldn't walk. The gift of faith had ignited from us to her!

A woman was healed of nerve deafness because the gift of faith spread across the auditorium!

The arm grew to full size and length, BUT THE HAND WAS STILL THE HAND OF A TWELVE-YEAR-OLD BOY! That didn't faze us one single bit. We were still operating under the supernatural anointing and power of the gift of faith, and as we commanded the hand to grow to normal size, that twelve-year-old hand unfolded like a rose to be the same size as the forty-year-old hand on the other arm.

Why?

Because the gift of faith fell sovereignly that night! And two ordinary people became supernatural people of God! And so can you!

By Charles

God speaks to his people in many different ways. Sometimes when he speaks, it is in such a seemingly ordinary, human way that we hardly know it is God. Everyone has at one time or another wondered if it was God speaking, or just the thought of the human involved. The gift of faith operates differently! It will come through God speaking or through revelation knowledge! This can occur when you are praying for the sick, whether it is one or one hundred, and suddenly you very simply "know" that the healing will take place.

In the case of Jeffie, it is difficult to tell how God spoke, because we were so new in the operation of the gifts of the Spirit. There was a sudden moment when we had the positive assurance in our hearts that we were to take off the braces. To remove braces without positively hearing from God is sometimes dangerous; it should only be done when you have that "faith assurance." Presumption can do harm — faith can heal!

There are times when the gift of faith and the word of knowledge will operate hand-in-hand, although they do not always do so. When God gives a word of knowledge, which is through a word or a feeling in the body, it can be relied on to be 100% accurate; however, this is different than the operation of, and the receiving of, the gift of faith. When you are operating completely in the

Spirit, both of these can be relied on completely; however, the gift of faith accompanying a word of knowledge will make an electrifying charge of faith-without-a--doubt surge through your spirit. Nothing that you can feel, but a heart knowledge of what is happening!

Several years ago while we were ministering in El Paso, Texas, God spoke to both of us at exactly the same moment and told us we were to have a miracle service on the following Tuesday night. We had never had a miracle service in our entire life! We had just received the baptism with the Holy Spirit shortly before this, but we KNEW it was God who spoke! We boldly announced what God had spoken to our hearts because the gift of faith had dropped on us and we knew that we could depend on God doing miracles. There was no doubt, no hesitation, no holding back, no questioning, no nothing, except boldness to proclaim what God was going to do.

The gift of faith is not in operation at all times, and is not something for which you can "pray through." It is something that God sovereignly drops as we wills, at a specific time and for a specific purpose. We should always be sensitive to the Spirit of God, so that we do not pass up some of the wonderful things of the supernatural that God has for us. This gift does not operate for healings only, but for many other areas of our lives. The gift of faith will give us unusual daring and confidence in business dealings. The gift of faith was in operation when we married without knowing each other, only that God told us to be married! (See MY LOVE AFFAIR WITH CHARLES).

Peter operated in the gift of faith when he walked on the water. Jesus operated in the gift of faith when he turned water into wine — he also operated in the gift of miracles simultaneously.

There have been times when the gift of faith drops on people we have prayed for and it does not drop on us. This is just as valid as if it had dropped on us, and we are just as surprised at the response and behavior of individuals as they are surprised at us!

A lady came forward one night in Minneapolis for healing of a compound fracture. She had broken her leg one week prior to the service, the doctor had put her in a cast and told her it would be six weeks before it could be removed. We ministered to her in the prayer line by simply laying hands on the cast and commanding the leg to be healed.

The gift of faith fell sovereignly upon her! She was so positive that God had healed her that as soon as she arrived home that night she soaked the cast off in the bathtub! The next night she came back to testify, and what a testimony she gave! Not in words, but in action! She jumped up and down on the leg as hard as she could to prove she was totally healed!

We did not operate in the gift of faith. BUT SHE DID!

HOWEVER!!! The next day we were in Denver and before the service a girl about thirteen years old walking on crutches, came up to the book table. Suddenly the gift of faith began to operate because when I saw her, I remembered what had happened just one night before! I KNEW SHE WOULD BE HEALED! I don't know how I knew, but I knew! I questioned her to see if she wanted to be healed before or after the service! At first she said she would wait until after the service, but then she said, "No, I want to be healed BEFORE the service!"

I simply ran my hands over the foot and ankle and said, "In the name of Jesus, bones, I command you to be healed." Notice that I spoke directly to the bones. My spirit was leaping because of the gift of faith, so I said, "Test it to see what God has done!"

She stepped on it, gently and gingerly, and a shock-ed look came on her face! She pressed down a little harder, then a little harder, and soon she began to cry with joy! She came on the stage before the whole church that morning, and again that night, to dance before the Lord and tell of his mighty act! Was I surprised? No, because the gift of faith was in operation; therefore, I could tell her to act without a moment's doubt! I'll tell you one thing, though, we are thrilled and excited every time God does a miracle!

Along the same lines, I had spoken at our City of Light Christian Center church service, when the anointing of God came on me strongly in ever-increasing power. Frances received the gift of faith and ran to the front. She said, "Charles, tell EVERYONE who needs healing to come forward right now!"

In my spirit I KNEW that anyone I touched would be healed. The first one was a woman who had come from California with a severe knee problem which the doctors could not diagnose. She was discouraged because it seemed as though nothing could be done. I was so full of the gift of faith, I just touched her knee, and she threw the crutches as high as she could and started running — free from pain!

Next I ran to a twelve-year-old girl nearby who had fractured her foot and ankle the day before. Prior to the service, her mother had told us she could not even bear a tiny amount of pressure on it without crying. Even with pain pills, she was in excruciating pain. She was also on crutches, but when I simply touched her foot and said, "Be healed in the name of Jesus," I KNEW SHE WAS! Why? Because the gift of faith dropped on us after preaching the Word to the people!

The little girl hesitated to put her foot down, but finally she gingerly touched the carpet. A look of surprise came over her face! Then she pressed a little more, and a little more, and a little more, until suddenly she said, "Mama, it doesn't hurt any more!" Mama quickly took off the "half" cast, and the little girl took off on a run. She ran completely around the big circular dome and that night she came back wearing tennis shoes, playing as normally as anyone.

Her mother came up to us at the evening service because when they had gotten home her husband was very upset about the whole thing and said, "Those Pentecostals have just psyched you out. You didn't get healed!" As a result, he was insistent that the little girl go back to the doctor to have it checked, and the mother did not know what to do.

She said, "Will it show a lack of faith if I take her back to the doctor?"

Frances said, "He won't believe you. He won't believe me, but HE WILL BELIEVE THE DOCTOR, so go ahead, because God's healings will stand the test."

The next morning the mother took the little girl to the doctor. The little girl was so excited, she just blurted out, "Doctor, Jesus healed my ankle yesterday at church!"

The doctor said, "We'll see about that!" He X-rayed it, and after examining it said, "You are right, because you have had a miracle!"

Later, the unsaved husband was heard telling his sister, "Do you know what happened yesterday? God healed our little girl's foot while she was at church!"

Jesus heals so that people will believe that he is the Son of God, and is the only way into eternal life. Glory!

Be aware of the gift of faith at all times, so that when the glory begins to fall, you'll be right there!

Peter and John had the gift of faith drop on them when they went up to the temple one day. The man who had probably begged alms of Jesus was there, and it would have been easy for them to think, "Jesus didn't heal this man, so why should we try?" But they didn't! Why? Because the gift of faith came upon them, and without any doubt, as Peter fastened his eyes upon him with John, said, *"Look on us ..."* Then Peter said, *"Silver and gold have I none; but such as I have give I thee: In the name of Jesus Christ of Nazareth rise up and walk"* (Acts 3:4,6).

This was an illustration of the working of the gift of faith. The same thing can happen to you, so BE ALERT!

You don't even have to be in a church service when the gift of faith falls. During lunch time one day, three of us remained in an auditorium where we were holding a meeting. We looked up and saw a couple entering, pushing a little girl in a tiny wheel chair. The gift of faith came upon both of us at the same time!

We went directly to them and inquired as to what the problem was. They told us the child had been attacked by a disease which caused the muscles to become useless. Already she could not move her legs, and it was beginning in her arms.

A friend had been to our services the night before and saw Jesus healing the sick. She called them and said, "You've got to take Belinda! She'll be healed, I know she will!" Their faith ignited, and suddenly they believed that if they could get the forty miles to the service, their little girl could be healed!

We said to the child, "Do you believe God will heal you?" Without any doubt, she instantly said, "I HAVE FAITH IN GOD!"

We said, "Then, IN THE NAME OF JESUS, STAND UP AND WALK!"

She shot out of the wheel chair as though she was a rocket taking off, and FELL FLAT ON HER FACE!

Did our faith fall flat with her? NO! Why? Because God dropped the gift of faith on us!

We picked her up off the floor, stood her on her feet, and said, "NOW, WALK, IN JESUS' NAME!"

She took one step, AND SHE DIDN'T FALL DOWN!

She took another step, AND SHE DIDN'T FALL DOWN! Pretty soon she started walking all over the place, and her parents took the wheel chair back to the car so she wouldn't even see it again.

That afternoon she danced for Jesus on the stage of the auditorium!

... And there was an interesting postscript to the healing!

Five years previously, the wife of a Christian book store owner in Albuquerque came to a meeting, with the same incurable disease little Belinda had. She was on crutches with her legs dangling like they didn't have any bones in them. They looked like a rubber doll's legs.

Bobbie was the first one at the meeting, and sat right in the middle of the front row. When she came in, she said, "I believe when you pray for me, I'll be healed!" And while we were making preparations for the meeting, she kept saying excitedly, "Tonight's my night to be healed!"

She came up on crutches and when we prayed, she fell under the power. She said that Frances threw the crutches across the room and said, "You'll never need them again!" All we remember is she looked so pathetic on the floor, struggling to get up with those legs of rubber. Finally she made it, and although she was walking, she didn't look like she was healed. But we look not with the natural eyes, but with eyes of faith.

She had come to the meeting to tell us of her healing, little realizing there would be a little girl there with the same disease. She said, "The only thing I haven't been able to do is dance," so Charles said, "Come on, let's dance right now!" And she and Charles danced before the Lord as all of us praised and worshiped God for her healing.

Many people wonder if God's healings last! Of course they do! Bobbie walks perfectly today!

There are times when you need to heal without the gift of faith, but when those beautiful, holy times come and God literally dumps the gift of faith on you, step out without a doubt and ACT QUICKLY AND WITH FULL CONFIDENCE!

When the gift of faith is fully given, you step out of

the dimension of the human limitations and step into the dimension of Almighty God!

"For with God nothing shall be impossible" (Luke 1:37).

"... *AND NOTHING SHALL BE IMPOSSIBLE UNTO YOU"* (Matt. 17:20).

CHAPTER 17

CREATIVE MIRACLES

By Charles

God does creative miracles! He makes physical things out of things that do not exist. He said, *"Let there be light . . ."* and light came into being (Gen. 1:3). *"And God CREATED great whales, and every living creature that moveth . . ."* (Gen. 1:21).

God extended himself, with all his powers, into us through Jesus, so his same power through us can CREATE parts for bodies which become defective. When you buy a car or an appliance, you need to consider the availability of new parts when the old ones wear out. God loves us and cares for us much more than a car manufacturer cares for his cars, so he provides a means of replacing defective or worn-out parts for our bodies.

You, too, can call into being those things which do not exist, using the power of God in the name of Jesus!

The Bible tells us that God *"quickeneth the dead, and calleth those things which be not as though they were"* (Rom. 4:17).

According to The Living Bible: *"God will accept all people in every nation who trust God as Abraham did. And this promise is from God himself, who makes the dead live again and speaks of future events with as much certainty as though they were already past"* (Rom. 4:17 TLB).

Shortly after Frances and I received the baptism with the Holy Spirit, I was reading the Living Bible and the Holy Spirit made a scripture come alive to me! *"Jesus now returned to the Sea of Galilee, and climbed a hill and sat there. And a vast crowd brought him their lame, blind, maimed, and those who couldn't speak, and many others, and laid them before Jesus, and he healed them all. What a spectacle it was! Those who hadn't been able to say a word before were talking excitedly, and those with missing arms and legs had new ones; the crippled were walking and jumping around, and those who had been blind were gazing about them! The crowd just marveled, and praised the God of Israel"* (Matt. 15:29-31 TLB).

I went to my CPA office after reading that story and couldn't get it off my mind. I called Frances and said, "God is going to do creative miracles in our ministry; he is going to grow out limbs that aren't there! We are going to see real legs grow where wooden legs are now! My faith was ignited as we talked about actually experiencing such phenomenal things as that!

About a month or two later, we were in Florida at a non Spirit-filled church when the pastor said we would have to conclude our service by 9 PM because his people would walk out if we held them too long.

God began displaying his amazing power, and somewhere around 11 PM the glory of God fell on a fourteen-year-old boy. We said, "What would you like Jesus to do for you?"

He stuck out his hand and showed us a missing thumb, cut off at the back joint, and said he wanted God to grow him a new thumb!

Hallelujah! Did we ever get excited! After just having discovered that scripture, God was giving us an opportunity to put it into practice, and to call into being that which did not exist!

By this time, the audience was wild with excitement as they were watching the spectacular miracles God was doing, one right after the other. They were no longer sitting! They were not only standing on the pews, but some were standing on the backs of pews, holding onto the ones standing on the pews! We didn't even know what the gift of faith was, but we knew what God had said to us about growing new parts!

We had him hold out both hands so we could see the difference, and we began commanding the thumb to grow in Jesus' name! We were almost shouting, "GROW! GROW! GROW!"

Suddenly, it began to grow! You could see the end of it moving out slowly alongside the other thumb.

The people were screaming! And so were we! Because God was re-enacting his first earthly miracles of creation!

In a matter of just a few moments, maybe a minute, the thumb was full-grown, just like the other! It had normal knuckles, and a place for a thumbnail, but there was no nail on it. Expectantly we said, "Let's ask God for a thumbnail!" Hallelujah! Why not? God is in that kind of creative part-making business.

With about seventy-five people looking, we boldly commanded a thumbnail to grow, in Jesus' name! And it did! We watched it as it slowly grew out, but were really surprised when it continued growing past the end of the thumb! It curved over the end and back down the underside of the thumb, like a talon! Around it was a soft blue glow. We all excitedly discussed the unusual way it had formed, and looked closely at it for several minutes!

Good news travels fast, and the next morning many were waiting for the boy to come to church and were excited to see what God had done. The new thumb was perfect! BUT THERE WAS NO EVIDENCE OF THE THUMBNAIL —JUST THE PLACE FOR IT! We couldn't understand what had happened, because so many of us had actually seen it there.

As we thought about it, we recalled visions from God

where a blue glow surrounded the person or object made visible in the spirit, but not physically. We can only assume that this was a vision of God, where he let about seventy-five people see the same thing — in the spirit!

Shortly after this, our grandson brought a little neighbor boy over to his house one night while we were there. The boy had one foot about a half inch shorter than the other. We commanded it to grow out, but saw no evidence of change. However, the next morning the boy came running over, exclaiming that both feet were the same length and the same size! The leg which had been approximately one-half the size of the full-size leg, had filled out during the night and was also a normal leg!

In Wisconsin several years ago a thirteen-year-old girl came to a miracle service expecting a BIG miracle. She had been to an orthodontist because of crooked, overlapping, protruding teeth. They were badly covered with tartar, and her gums were soft and bleeding. The fees for corrective work were so great that the family could not afford to have the much-needed work done.

While we were worshiping God and praising Jesus in song, the little girl turned to her mother and exclaimed, "Mother, my teeth are moving!" Her mother got so excited she didn't even stop to look! She just said, "Get up there as fast as you can!"

The girl ran to the front, but the glory of God was so upon her that before she got on the stage, she fell under the power of God, and lay there for about thirty minutes.

When she got up, her teeth were so perfect that Frances said they looked like an ear of corn with perfectly straight rows! To me it looked like God had created a full set of new teeth out of heavenly pearls! They were perfectly shaped and her gums were beautiful and healthy! We could hardly believe what we were seeing!

We asked if there was a dentist present, and a young man who had driven four hours to get there ran up to us.

When he looked in her mouth, he said, "I have never seen such a perfect and beautiful set of teeth in my life!"

God had done another creative miracle, and, just as he said in Genesis 1:25, after he had made the beast and the cattle and other creeping things after his kind, *"And God saw that IT WAS GOOD."*

The gift of the word of knowledge is always exciting to experience, but especially when used in conjunction with a creative miracle! One night during a miracle service, my gums and face felt like I had been to a dentist and had a shot of Novocain to deaden the pain. I recognized this as a signal from God that he was healing someone with a tooth problem. When I announced this to the audience, five people came forward. God had filled the cavities in the teeth of two of them; he had healed two with abscesses; and the fifth one said she had been to the dentist that day, THAT HE HAD DEADENED HER MOUTH WITH NOVOCAIN, had filled two teeth and prepared the other three for more work the next day! God had filled the other three teeth perfectly and the dead feeling had left her face! Glory to God who does the impossible today —creative miracles for the masses!

While we were on that same trip, a filling came out of one of Frances' teeth. She showed it to me, I examined it and threw it into a waste basket. When we returned home, she went to the dentist to have the filling replaced. As she was parking, she said, "God, you filled all those other teeth. Why do I have to waste all this time going to a dentist to have mine filled?"

The technician sat her in the dentist chair and said, "What is the problem?" Frances said, "The filling came out of a tooth."

The technician examined it, and said, "Which tooth do you mean?" Frances showed her again, and then again, but the technician could not locate where the filling had come out! She called the dentist in and they repeated the same routine, and he could find no missing filling. God is a great and loving God of surprises! How we praise him!

During a visit to Australia, a television station sent a crew to cover one of our miracle services. The very first thing they wanted to know was, "What is a miracle?" They had never seen God do miracles, and were excited about what was going to happen, even if they were not Christians.

We explained to them that there were many healings that you could not see or photograph, but there were certain types of miracles that you could actually see while they were happening. We told them to feel at liberty to interview the individuals beforehand, during and after the healing, and even photograph it as it took place.

"How well he knew their thoughts! But he said to the man with the deformed hand, 'Come and stand here where everyone can see'" (Luke 6:8 TLB). Jesus called into being something that did not exist, and had even told them that it would happen before the healing took place.

The Australian miracle service was underway! The cameras were rolling. We had everyone measure their arms, and then the ushers selected a few from the audience who had enough difference in the length of their arms to be seen from the stage. The first one was a simple adjustment, and it was accomplished very quickly!

The next person was a lady whose left arm was about two inches shorter than the right. We asked her what caused the arm to be short. Her reply shocked us, because she said the doctor had removed about two inches of bone from the arm!

Right on national television I looked up to God and said, "God, you had better be here for this one!" God had better be there for every miracle, or they won't happen, but in this case I wanted to make sure he was there!

But God is faithful and wants to demonstrate his power so people will believe that he is a living God! As we commanded that arm to grow, it did so — at just the right speed for all of Australia to see God in action on a television screen!

God had put in two inches of bone, marrow, tissue, nerves, muscles, and whatever else it takes to extend an arm two inches. He had done a creative miracle as we commanded the arm to grow in Jesus' name! If that creative miracle had happened in the synagogue two thousand years ago, it would possibly have been in Luke 6:8, or some other exciting scripture!

One Thursday night in Houston, we commanded a new part to be formed in a lady, and exactly one month later she returned and reported she went to the hospital the next Monday for surgery after we had prayed for her and received an interesting diagnosis from the doctor: "You won't need surgery because there seems to be a NEW uterus!" If God can put a star into a fixed position, he can put a new uterus into one of his children!

One night in Oregon a man came for healing who had one lung which had been collapsed by a surgeon seven years before. We laid our hands on him, commanded a new lung to appear, and commanded his breathing to be normal. The next morning he told us excitedly that he was filling that lung with air as easily as the other. We talked with him several times later, and he said it was great to have two perfect lungs! Hallelujah!

One night the Spirit of God led us to ask how many had never seen someone fall in the Spirit, or go under the power. Over half of the audience said they had not, so we asked for twenty volunteers who wanted a touch from God to come forward!

We had felt led to ask this question because we had prayed for someone at the very beginning of the service. When that person fell under the power, a gasp went up all over the audience, so we knew this was something that not everyone present had seen before. It didn't surprise us when half the audience arose to come forward.

There was a limited amount of ministering room, so we lined up about twenty across the front of the audience, and then we touched each one on the forehead gently and simply said, "Jesus, touch them!" Every single one of them fell backwards to the floor, and a surprising thing happened! Normally people get right back up, but this time they all continued to stay right there.

We finally started singing and praising God, because momentarily it looked as though they were going to stay there all night! Suddenly a young woman on the floor started laughing hilariously! She put her hand over her mouth, but couldn't stop! Soon a dignified business-man next to her on the floor did exactly the same thing! First he put his hand over his mouth, but before long, he was laughing almost hysterically, completely unable to stop. Then another, and another, until it wasn't long before all those under the power and the entire audience were doing exactly the same thing! They were all laughing hilariously as wave after wave of holy laughter spread over everyone!

Finally, the first young lady who had gone down under the power got up, still laughing energetically, ran over to another lady, and started beating her on the shoulder! We knew she wasn't angry, but couldn't undertand what she was doing! When we finally got her settled down so she could talk, she explained that her aunt had "forced" her to come to the meeting against her desire. She had one arm which had atrophied because of an incurable disease, and she could not even lift it. She was a nurse, so she couldn't work because of this. She was demonstrating to her aunt by hitting her that God had healed her, because she was laughing so hard she couldn't talk!

While everyone was still laughing, a man said to his wife whose glasses had fallen off when she went under the power, "Honey, your eye got healed! It isn't crossed any more!"

A sixteen-year-old girl was watching all this, and while she was laughing, she began to feel movement in her foot. She had always had to buy two pair of shoes, because she had one foot smaller than the other, and right in front of her eyes, the smaller foot grew to the same length as the other one! Hallelujah!

But the biggest surprise came the next morning when a lady who had been working at the book table reported that during the period of holy laughter, God had restored a breast which had been partially removed in surgery! Hallelujah!

We were sharing this with Dr. Lester Sumrall shortly after that and said, "We didn't know there was power in holy laughter." He said, "THERE IS POWER IN ANYTHING THAT IS HOLY!"

What had happened? What methods did God use to heal all these people and scores of others during that one night of real glory?

The WORD OF KNOWLEDGE caused us to call them forward.

The HOLY LAUGHTER was given by the Spirit as a healing balm.

The GIFTS OF HEALING were in operation.

We LAID HANDS ON THEM.

The divine presence of the HOLY SPIRIT brought power to heal.

FAITH ignited among the people as God began to allow his power to flow supernaturally.

How do you heal the sick in a situation like that? All we can say is when the Spirit is moving, move right with him!!!

By Frances

We all think that the most exciting healing that ever happens is the one that happens to us, and I'm no different than you. I want to share what God did in my life in the way of a creative miracle!

Some seven years ago I desperately needed a BIG healing. I had an enlarged heart with a hole in it. My blood pressure was 225/140 after medication! I have a very high pain tolerance, and that is why, if I ever do get sick, I am unaware of the fact that I actually am sick. I totally believe in God and his healing power, so I forget to notice some symptoms that might occasionally come upon me.

I cannot help but think of how many times my blood pressure had skyrocketed and given me such headaches that I thought my head was going to blow off, and yet I still did not even think there was anything wrong with me. I would say to Charles, "Honey, I have a horrible headache, and you KNOW I never have head-aches!" Then one day Charles answered me and said, "Honey, did it ever dawn on you how many times you've been saying that lately?"

The week that Bob and Joan were to be married, the devil took a real poke at me, and I had gone to bed because I had more pain than I could possibly stand. My head felt like it was bursting open. I had been in bed for 48 hours when Charles got mad at the devil! He jumped on top of the bed, and I have never seen Charles speak with such great authority in my entire life. He really yelled at the devil! God had just spoken to him to take authority over the heart, and when God speaks to Charles, he acts with great power and faith.

A technician was taking my blood pressure, and when Charles took authority over the heart, he spoke to it and said words to this effect: "Devil, you take your hands off my sweetheart! Heart, in the name of Jesus, I take authority and dominion over you, and I command you to reduce to normal size! Blood pressure, I command you to go down to normal, in the name of Jesus! Hole in the heart, I command you in the name of Jesus to be healed, RIGHT NOW!"

Charles said he was speaking to an enemy he hated who was attacking his beloved and he really meant business. He wasn't just saying words!

And God did a supernatural miracle! He brought the blood pressure down to 140/80 in a matter of twelve minutes, and it has remained there to this very day! My horrible headache completely disappeared, and I have never had one since then!

The most exciting thing, however, is the fact that when X-rays were made after this, there was no more hole in the heart, nor was it enlarged. As a matter of fact, the doctor showed me the X-ray made before the healing, and the one after the healing, and said, "Frances, you have the heart of a sixteen-year old girl!"

Charles is a very strong, but sweet, mild-mannered person, but he scared me so that night when he jumped up on the bed and started yelling and pointing at my heart that I was afraid not to get healed! I have never seen Charles the real tiger he was that night, but the gift of faith really fell on him, and God did a creative miracle! Glory to God! It's not how loud you yell, but it is important that you believe in your heart and speak with authority because that is the way Jesus said to do it.

We give God all the praise and honor because that new heart is what has kept me running all these years for the Lord!

Let's look back over these examples and scriptures and see "how to heal the sick" to obtain a creative miracle.

There are times when we simply ask God for a new part for a body, and he responds. We don't limit God in any way, because he has demonstrated hundreds of times that he heals in many different and unique ways, and we are astounded at the ease with which he does it. Jesus did it. The disciples did it. As you see by these few examples, Frances and Charles did it. And so can you!

There are times when we command a part to be formed in a body, and suddenly something appears that was not there before! *"Through faith we understand that the worlds were framed by the word of God, so that things which are seen were not made of things which do appear"* (Heb. 11:3). Generally we also lay hands on those to whom we are ministering. Most of the time they fall under the power.

Just as God speaks things into existence, we can do the same because he lives in us by the power of the Holy Spirit.

We must believe that we have the power of God and the authority of Jesus to apply this power.

We must believe that we are doing the will of the Father; that we are doing it for his pleasure and his glory.

We must be willing to walk on spiritual water and never be concerned with what others think about us.

We must act upon what the Word of God declares that others have done, and believe that *"... He that believeth on me, the works that I do shall he do also; and greater works that these shall he do; because I go unto my Father. And whatsoever ye shall ask in my name, that will I do, that the Father may be glorified in the Son"* (John 14:12,13).

We must not let our trust in God falter when we start toward a miracle — keep going no matter how little you understand about what God is doing; move rapidly when the Spirit is doing unusual things.

Operate in a combination of the gifts of the Spirit, because they are the tools which God gives us to perform the supernatural.

"Expect God to act!" (Ps. 42:11 TLB).

Watch for opportunities to glorify God and Jesus by doing those things which show that Jesus is the way, the truth, and the life, so that people will want to serve God.

Be bold! Speak with authority; operate in love! *"Faith ... worketh by love"* (Gal. 5:6).

Live like you really believe you are the body of Christ! If you actually believe that you are the dwelling place of God's Holy Spirit, that you are endued with HIS power, that Jesus lives in you, then you should be willing to DO THE IMPOSSIBLE just for him!

Don't limit your healing methods to prayer, or the way someone else has done it. Jesus didn't! He was original in almost every act he did.

CALL INTO BEING PARTS WHICH DO NOT EXIST!

CHAPTER 18
GROWING OUT ARMS AND LEGS

By Frances

There are many common, ordinary, unusual, and unique ways to heal the sick. God has told us only a few of them, and we never attempt to limit God and put him in a box. He surprises us constantly because almost every time we minister healing, or teach on healing the sick, God shows us something new, so that adds to our knowledge and God multiplies the number of healings.

It is somewhat like developing an automobile. It would have been hard to invent an automobile if a wheel had not been invented years before. They already had the wheel so all they had to do was get a motor and hook it up to the wheel! It is the same with healing! You learn a little and you add that to what you already know. Then you learn a little more, and you add a little more knowledge. If you will just keep on healing the sick, you will keep learning more about how to heal.

When do you heal the sick? When you feel like it? No! When you think there is a special anointing on you? No! You lay hands when there is an opportunity. Whether your ministry is preaching, ministering salvation or the baptism with the Holy Spirit, healing, casting out devils, operating in the supernatural gifts of the spirit, or whatever, it is always your job to use the tools

God gives you at any particular moment.

If you will let God work through you, and have the freedom to do things even if you don't have any idea as to whether you will succeed or not, and you just jump out of the boat and start walking on the water like Peter did, you will be absolutely amazed that God will honor that act of faith! You literally have to learn to walk on water spiritually to heal the sick. When you are willing to step out of the boat, Jesus will be there.

In the charismatic world, growing out arms and legs is very common, and is done in big and small meetings all over the world.

The very first time I ever saw this type of miracle done, I will have to be honest with you, IT TURNED ME OFF! I really thought the evangelist was pulling some kind of a trick. Probably the thing that influenced me the most was the fact that it seemed like everyone in the audience had a short arm or leg, and I knew this wasn't possible! Since then, we have found out that over eighty percent of the world's population have back problems, and this is one of the greatest single ailments in the world!

However, about a month after that, God brought the same evangelist to Houston, and we were sitting on the platform with him when a lady came up who had an arm about three or four inches short, and it grew out RIGHT UNDER MY NOSE! I didn't doubt any more!

Right after this, we met a Spirit-filled chiropractor, Dr. Jack Herd, of Harrisburg, Pennsylvania, and he told us about the percentage of back problems, and this began to make us think that there was some great healing potential from growing out an arm or a leg, so we began to experiment. We thought, "If it will work for one evangelist, it will work for us!" In the beginning, we really yelled loud and long, and prayed and prayed, but little by little we began to see results! The growing out of arms was not just a physical miracle that you could see, but it was God's way of adjusting or healing a back problem.

One night we had eight backs healed all at one time! When people began telling us how the pain left their backs the minute their arms or legs grew out, we began to sit up and take notice of what God was doing, and we began to appreciate more and more the benefits and magnitude of this miracle!

Cowboy Ralph McRae had three smashed discs in his back when he came to his first miracle service. I pointed him out in the balcony and said, "Your back has just been healed!" Instantly he felt the warm power of the Holy Spirit go down all the way through his spine, and he was totally healed! Up to that time he had been wearing a "corset" to ride, but he has not had to wear one since the night of his healing. However, another very interesting thing happened!

He was so wound up after the service that he couldn't go to sleep, so he started to read the Bible. He put on his glasses which he had worn for 31 years but HE COULDN'T SEE! Alarmed, he said, "God, you didn't heal my back just to let me go blind, did you?" He took the glasses off to clean them and discovered his vision was perfect WITHOUT THE GLASSES! God had healed his eyes at the same time he healed his back.

We didn't associate the two healings until God began to show us a relationship between back healings and other healings. Could the back adjustment have relieved an optical nerve or adjusted an eye muscle to bring back the vision?

Another night a man came for prayer who had been in an accident about thirty-seven years previously, in which his back had been severely injured. Someone who was with him suggested that he ought to have his ear prayed for at the same time because he was stone-deaf in one ear. Charles asked him what caused the deafness and he said, "It happened the same time my back was injured!"

Normally, Charles would have put his fingers in his ears and commanded the deaf spirit to come out, or he would have said, "Open, in the name of Jesus," but before he could do that, God clearly spoke to him and said, "Grow out his leg and he can hear!" Talk about confounding the wise with foolish things — who ever heard of growing a leg out to heal a deaf ear? We certainly had not, but Charles was obedient.

He said, "Sit down; God said to grow your leg out and you can hear!" I'm glad he didn't have time to think that over because he might have thought Charles was crazy. Charles measured his legs and one was about three inches shorter than the other. He commanded the back to be healed, and COMMANDED HIS MUSCLES, NERVES, AND TENDONS TO BE ADJUSTED, and his leg to grow.

The leg grew quickly to full length, and Charles tested his ear. HE COULD HEAR PERFECTLY! He went all over the church telling everyone he could hear with his deaf ear. He was so excited about hearing that he forgot to check his back for about an hour, and then discovered his back was healed, too! Apparently the injury had pinched or damaged a nerve to his ear and caused nerve deafness.

This was a new insight for us into God's healing world! Just about a week later a young lady came to be healed of total deafness in one ear. She said it was a dead nerve, so Charles checked her arms. One was nearly an inch short, so he used the same commands he did with the man. Her arm grew out and instantly she could hear perfectly.

Hundreds have been healed this same way since we discovered there is obviously a connection between nerve deafness and back problems!

Since growing out arms and legs seems so common-place to us, we overlooked the vast field of healings that belongs in this type of healing. God has been revealing more and more miracles relating to back, muscle, and nerve adjustments.

We were in Washington recently, and a man brought a thirteen-year-boy to Ralph (the cowboy) for healing of bed-wetting. As Ralph began to pray, God spoke to him and said, "Grow out his leg and he'll be healed!" This really shocked Ralph, but instead of praying as he had originally planned, he sat the boy down on a chair, measured his legs, and discovered one was approximately two inches shorter than the other. The leg grew out.

We want you to think about that healing. Isn't it logical that this could cause pressure on the kidneys or bladder? We talked to doctors and chiropractors since then and they agree that this could very easily cause bed-wetting!

We know without having medical knowledge, that nerves and muscles are used in a body to effect normal functions, so if a nerve or muscle is bound or pinched, it can cause a body defect or malfunction. This could cause a bladder or kidney problem.

We have talked to medical doctors and chiropractors, not to learn how to be doctors because we are not qualified for that, nor do we intend to practice medicine, but to discuss some of these ways God is healing by back, muscle, nerve or other adjustments.

A chiropractor friend really got excited when we spent some time talking with him about the specific ways God has healed through this method. He pointed out to us some of their profession's findings relating to spinal misalignments. One of the things he told us was that the nervous system controls and coordinates all organs and structures of the human body, and that misalignments of spinal vertebrae and discs may cause irritation to the nervous system and affect the structures, organs, and functions which may result in the conditions we were mentioning and many others.

For example, he related that what is labeled verte-
bra Number 2C, second from top of the spine, controls
the eyes, optic nerves, auditory nerves, sinuses, mastoid
bones, tongue, and forehead. We don't know whether all
doctors agree with this or not, but we have noticed that
when God makes an adjustment in upper or lower
spinal areas, hundreds of backs have been healed, and
other healings such as Cowboy Ralph's eyes occurred
when the back was healed. We feel that we should take
notice of what God is doing through adjustments, and
what doctors and chiropractors already know.

This same chiropractor said that we would probably
be amazed if we knew how many problems which have
not even shown up yet, are prevented by backs being
adjusted in our meetings.

One thing we know for sure is that our ignorance of
what takes place when God adjusts a back, muscles,
nerves, or whatever else he does, does not result in our
making a bunch of damaging mistakes, because we are
not doing it — God is!

By Charles

You may have never seen an arm or a leg grow out.
If not, you're in for a real treat! One of the most exciting
miracles you will ever see is to watch the power of God
actually move a part of the body, right in front of your
eyes. This is also perhaps the simplest and most common-
ly performed of all miracles. It is tremendous to convince
a sinner or a person who has not yet received the
baptism with the Holy Spirit of the reality of the power
of a living God who has not forgotten how to heal the
sick.

You might want to try it on yourself! Stand up straight, put your feet together so that your toes are even, and look straight forward. Extend your arms in front of you with the palms facing each other, about a half-inch apart, and then push or stretch your arms straight out as far as you can.

While your arms are stretched, bring your hands tightly together and hold them together until you bend your elbows so that you can see the ends of your fingers. If the length of your arms is uneven, the fingers on your long arm will come out farther than those on your short arm. Now you are ready to grow out your own arm. Stretch your arms out in front of you again, letting your hands lightly touch each other, but don't hold them tightly together.

You might want to say something like this, "Arm, in the name of Jesus, I command you to grow. Spine, muscles, nerves, ligaments and tendons, be adjusted in the name of Jesus." Then say, "Thank you, Father, I believe it is done," and stand there for a few moments and watch the miracle as it grows! You should see the short arm grow to equal the length of the other, and maybe even feel the adjustment.

Now do it to someone else!

If you want to try it on legs, have a person sit erect in a straight chair and stick their feet forward. You can often see the adjustment needed by looking at the bottoms of the shoes, or by putting your thumbs on the ankle bones. Hold the feet lightly in your hands and then command the back to align itself and the muscles, nerves and tendons to move into place and command the short leg to grow in the name of Jesus, and by the power of the Holy Spirit. You do all the work, and God gets all the glory! Generally if there is an upper back or neck problem, the arms will need adjusting, and if it is a lower back problem, the legs will be uneven. Check your back, or the back of the person to whom you are ministering, by bending it, and see if it didn't get healed when the arm or leg grew out. There are times when you need to adjust both the arms and legs.

Now you are ready to start being a common, ordinary, every-day miracle worker for Jesus, remembering that he is the Master and you are his servant to do HIS good will. It's fun and exciting to watch God's power do this type of healing, and it is a very effective witness to demonstrate God's power. Then, after God has done the miracle, don't forget the purpose: so that people will believe that Jesus is the way into eternal life. GET THEM SAVED! Or if they are saved, use this demonstration of the Spirit and of power for ministry as you teach on the baptism with the Holy Spirit, or for whatever purpose you feel impressed of the Spirit that is needed at the time. Remember, Jesus didn't come just to heal the sick; he came so that they would believe in his name and accept him and be saved!

We were talking one night to a young evangelist who works with college students. He walked into a fraternity house and said, "If you could have one wish, what would that wish be?" A young black student jumped up and said, "To have my two legs the same length!" He was wearing a built-up shoe, because one leg was about six inches shorter than the other. The young evangelist had just received the baptism shortly before this, but he sat the man down, and the leg grew a full six inches at his command! What a night of salvation it was for that fraternity! Miracles will do what words won't!

If there is a defective spinal disc or some other defective part, this must be divinely healed, or else surgery may be necessary. A medical doctor or chiropractor can often restore normal conditions by adjusting the segments of the spinal column. God can do this, too, and can do a much more permanent adjusting, because of the healing he can do at the same time. God often puts in new parts when needed, and he doesn't even charge extra for that service!

We have also discovered that the adjustment is not always in the spinal column, but is sometimes an adjustment of nerves, muscles, tendons, ligaments, or cartilages. A doctor might describe this better, but what it means is that parts need to be put back into their proper place by adjustments of some kind.

One lady had a jawbone which was not "hinged" right, and every time she bit down, it would pain her. This had been a life-long problem. I commanded the bone to align itself and the nerves and muscles and bones to be adjusted and released. The jawbone moved slightly and the pain left. She had a difficult time believing that a lifetime of pain left in a few seconds. God is so good!

We have commanded jaws to go into place when children have "overbites" and have seen jaws move into place and teeth line up. This hasn't worked every time, but we are going to keep trying every way we know to get as many as possible healed — all to the glory of God and in the name of Jesus!

A young lady came to one of our services who had never been to any kind of a healing service and was utterly astounded as possibly three or four hundred people were healed that night. She came to me after the service and said, "I looked at all of these people getting healed but I looked at all these people who have this power to heal, and almost all of them wear glasses. Since they can heal the sick, why do they wear glasses?"

I didn't really know what to say, but I later asked God why this is true!

One time Mel Tari, who wrote the book LIKE A MIGHTY WIND, visited our home. He shared about how God told him to go across a deep river and witness to some people, so he and his team walked over on top of the water! That was exciting to me. Hallelujah! I said,

"Are you still walking on water over there?"

He said, "No, it hasn't happened in seven years."

I said, "Why?"

He said, "They built a bridge upstream a little ways, and you do not have to walk on water; you can go to the bridge and get across."

I thought about that in relation to glasses. I don't really need to be healed, because with glasses, I have tremendous vision. I have perfect distant vision, but when I start to read, the words blur, so I wear glasses so that I can read. But why don't I get healed? Probably one of the big reasons is that I don't really need to be healed. If glasses had not been invented, and I couldn't see, I would get real serious with God!

We had not found an answer other than that one for eye problems, but recently while we were ministering in Canada, an ophthalmologist (eye doctor) excitedly asked Frances a question that may be leading to a tremendous advance in the number of eye healings we can see God do. He had heard us teach on growing out arms and legs, and how God was healing nerve deafness by a back adjustment. He said, "Do you know why so many people wear glasses?" Frances said she knew why she did — to see! He said, "Most people who need glasses have eye muscles of uneven length and the glasses are corrective for that. If God supernaturally adjusts the length of arms and legs, or adjusts muscles and nerves in a spine, why can't he do the same thing with eye muscles?"

What a spirit revelation this brought to us! We have just returned from a trip where we were on televison and had the opportunity to ask the viewing audience if they would help us in an experiment. We asked them to stand with their arms stretched out, and we prayed and commanded the eye muscles to adjust to the correct length for perfect vision for everyone who needed it!

Four telephone calls came back in immediately! One was a woman who was blind in one eye and had only ten percent vision in the other, and when she stood and received the prayer, she received sight in both eyes and could read the Bible!

A man reported his sight was gone in one eye, and during the prayer, his sight returned! Two other calls reporting eye healings were not quite so dramatic, but indicated that this could be the key unlocking the door to many eye healings.

We were on a plane on our way to California and were talking to a nurse. We began sharing about backs, and arms and legs growing out and she shared an interesting thought with us. She said whenever her mother felt like she was catching a cold, she immediately went to a chiropractor for an adjustment, and NEVER HAD A COLD! We decided that if the devil ever sneaks up on us again to attempt to put a cold on us, we will ask God to give us a good heavenly chiropractic treatment!

Another interesting miracle from growing out of arms: a singer came for prayer for lumps which had formed inside her throat. You could see fear that it was cancer written all over her face. I started to lay hands on her and command the lumps to leave, when a quiet word from God came as a thought. I tested her arms and sure enough they were uneven, so just as God had told me to do, I commanded the nerves and muscles to relax and go into place. Her arm grew out even, and I said, "Vicki, I dare you to find those lumps!" What joy she had when she could find no lumps!

We are going to share with you several other healings which God has done through the adjustments which often result from growing out arms and legs.

I woke up one morning with a charley horse in the top muscle of my shoulder. I simply stretched out my arms and commanded the muscle to relax, and one of the most beautiful experiences of my life happened. It was like the hand of Jesus released the muscle and the cramp gently faded away in a moment of time. The holy presence felt in my shoulder was as overwhelming as I believe the burning bush was to Moses!

All my life when I purchased a suit, the buttons did not match the button holes by about an inch because one shoulder was lower than the other. I had the tailor put a pad in the shoulder, and it was never as comfortable as the other shoulder. One day I just thought to God that I didn't really have to continue with that problem, and because he is so personal and real to us, I stood straight, squared my shoulders, and commanded them to be adjusted. I forgot about this until I purchased my next suit, and sure enough, the buttons matched the button holes perfectly. Oh, the beauty of God's personal love for his people.

The devil threw me at the floor one night and I fell unconscious. When I came to, my face pushed against the carpet floor, and I stood up, but my hand and elbow were in pain. The pain stayed with me a couple of months, especially as I twisted the elbow slightly. One day I was with a doctor friend and I asked him about this. He made a quick examination, and said this was a tennis elbow, and that he could give me a shot of cortisone to alleviate the pain. I thanked him, and said, "Now I know what to do." I went to my car, sat in the front seat, stretched forth my hands, and commanded the jammed tendon to stretch out to normal, and it did! I have never had a pain since then. The doctor had told me that when I fell, it jammed, or shortened, the tendon from my hand to my elbow. It's no wonder they call Jesus the GREAT PHYSICIAN!

We have seen muscle spasms stop, frozen elbows work normally, fatigue in the shoulder and neck muscles relax, headaches, pain in arms, hands, shoulders and other parts of the body be relieved, bodies go into traction as God adjusts the bones, muscles, and nerves or whatever else he does. All of these and scores of other healings and blessings are free gifts from God as his mighty power adjusts the right parts, and it is all IN THE NAME OF JESUS!

. God is showing the entire body of Christ, not just evangelists or ministers in a healing ministry, the simplicity of application of his awesome power so that the multitudes will not only receive healing, but will be freely giving to those around them, just as God has so freely given to us.

Thousands have been healed just in our ministry by this means of healing, and no doubt hundreds of thousands have received healing through others who have learned that they too can heal the sick. We feel in our spirits that God is saying that healings will soon be done by the millions throughout the world by people just like you!

You will never know until you try, but God is preparing the bride of Christ for that soon-coming return, and he will do it largely through the demonstration of his Spirit and his power. We want you to be a living part of this exciting move of God for the last days! Start growing out arms and legs!

CHAPTER 19
GO INTO ALL THE WORLD
... HEAL THE SICK

By Frances

"*As I was at this great height, I could behold the whole world. I watched these people as they were going to and fro over the face of the earth. Suddenly there was a man in Africa and in a moment he was transported by the Spirit of God, and perhaps he was in Russia, or China or America or some other place, and vice versa. All over the world these people went, and they came through fire, and through pestilence, and through famine. Neither fire nor persecution, nothing seemed to stop them.*"

"*As they marched forth in everything they did as the ministry of Christ in the end times, these people were ministering to the multitudes over the face of the earth. Tens of thousands, even millions seemed to come to the Lord Jesus Christ as these people stood forth and gave the message of the kingdom, of the coming kingdom, in this last hour.*"

Twenty years ago that exciting vision was given, and we see it coming to fulfillment today as mer and women are taking great steps forward to be among the multitudes who are sharing the Good News to the world!

In November of 1977 I had a dream, which for me is an unusual happening, because I normally do not dream. I dreamed that I was in a plane 37,000 feet in the air, which is nothing out-of-the-ordinary, because we fly all the time. There was something very unique about this ride, however, because I was standing in the OPEN doorway of the plane, with my knees bent, and my toes hanging over the doorway of the plane.

I heard a soft voice say, "Jump, I'll catch you!"

I looked down! Thirty-seven thousand feet in the air is a long way! Even in a dream, cold shivers went up and down my spine!

I knew it was God, and yet instantly I thought about the devil tempting Jesus. *"If you are the Son of God, jump off! For the scriptures say that God will send his angels to guard you and to keep you from crashing to the pavement below!"* (Luke 4:9TLB).

I looked down once more and it seemed even further this time!

Again, the voice said, "Jump, I'll catch you. Don't you trust me?"

It seemed as though I wrestled all night long, standing in the open door of the plane, and all night long the same voice kept saying over and over again, "Jump, I'll catch you. Don't you trust me?"

Every time I heard that voice I looked at how far above the earth we were, and 37,000 feet is a long way down! Yet in my heart I knew it was the voice of God, but I couldn't understand it. Suddenly I came to a conclusion because I thought, "What difference does it make? If it's the devil, I'll be splattered all over the ground, but I'll be in heaven instantly! And if it's God, and I'm disobedient, he might not ever talk to me again."

There was that sudden knowledge that I HAD to jump, so I let go and jumped right out into the unknown!

INSTANTLY I was on the earth! There was absolutely no time lapse between the jump and landing on the earth. There was no sensation of falling, no sensation of anything, just jumping, and being instantly there!

Once more I heard the soft, still voice of God say, "See, I told you that you could trust me!"

God had told us in a dream that we were going to take a giant step — a bigger step than we had ever taken before in our lives, but that he would be there at the end of the step to catch us!

We believe through that dream that God is telling the entire body of Christ to take a giant step and begin to do things they never dreamed of doing, and God will be there waiting for you!

God is calling you to take a giant step because he wants to make a giant out of you who will crush the devil under his very feet! And it's not going to happen because of ONE big giant, it's going to happen because of multiplied hundreds of thousands, perhaps even millions of Christians who are going to step out and begin laying hands on the sick, and healing them!

"And this is the miracle of it — this is the glorious miracle of it — those people would stretch forth their hands exactly as the Lord did, and it seemed as if there was this same liquid fire in their hands. As they stretched forth their hands, they said, 'According to my word, be thou made whole.' "

Twenty years ago those words were spoken! Note the similarity to the chapter entitled "A Vision is a Miracle" from the book we wrote in 1976 entitled IMPOSSIBLE MIRACLES:

FIVE YEARS AGO, I WOULDN'T HAVE BELIEVED THIS, BUT NOW I DO!

The final night of a Delightfully Charismatic Christian Walk Seminar in Calgary, Canada, was a night of power like we've never seen in our entire ministry.

Faith was at top level because of the seminar teachings. That night's subject was marriage, and as Charles was talking about honesty in marriage, I felt such a tremendous wave of power I nearly fell over. I grabbed the podium and looked over at Charles to see if he felt the same thing I did.

I couldn't believe my eyes!

Out of the ends of his fingers were shooting flames of blue fire about four inches long, and as I looked at them, God spoke to me and said, "The healing anointing is upon Charles. The first thirty people who reach the altar will be instantly healed!"

I had to interrupt Charles! The power was increasing to such an extent I knew God had something special! I repeated to the audience what God had said, and it looked like the entire auditorium turned upside down. I never saw sick and crippled people move so fast in my entire life!

As Charles ran off the stage to lay hands on them, the power of God was so strong they fell in waves as he ran through the crowd. When he was about half-way across the front of the auditorium, he raised his hands to touch some, and about thirty to forty people fell under the power at the same time. People began weeping all over the auditorium as they felt the power of God in a way they had never felt it before.

Bob and Joan were offstage at this particular moment, but they felt something supernatural come through the loudspeaker. Bob said, "I heard Frances, say, 'Get out of the way and let Charles through,' then I heard the word 'fire!' I came running out as fast as I could, wondering if there had been a bomb of some kind or other. There was —A HOLY GHOST BOMB! Charles was plowing through the crowd and people were falling all over the place!"

Joan said, "I kept hearing 'let him through, let him through, there's fire on his hands,' so I ran to the curtain at the back of the stage. The power of God was so strong it felt exactly like a solid wall of God's beautiful power, and I broke into tears, completely overcome by the overwhelming presence of God."

By this time Charles had gone almost across the auditorium, and the flames began to diminish, and finally they disappeared. He came back up onto the stage, and asked the people to raise their hands if they KNEW they were healed. More than 100 hands were raised, as God gave even more than he had promised.

It is impossible to explain how you feel in a moment like this. I was so awed by what I had seen and heard that I just stood there wondering what was going to happen next!

I didn't have to wait but just a few seconds and then I saw things I had never seen in my entire life. The Jubilee Auditorium is a large auditorium with two balconies, and an extremely high ceiling. As I looked out over the people, there appeared a huge dove with a wingspread of about fifty feet hovering on the left-hand side of the auditorium.

It was not white!

Instead, it was "like as of fire."

The dove looked exactly as if it had been carved right out of fire! It was red, orange and yellow!

I have never felt the awesome presence of God as I did at that moment, then a shocking thing began to happen!

The quills from the wings of the dove began flying out across the audience and landing on various people.

It looked like skyrockets exploding as the quills flew faster and faster across the auditorium.

God spoke again and said, "There is perversion in the sexual life of married couples here. There is adultery in marriages here, and I am sending the fire of my Holy Spirit to burn it out."

Men and women began weeping as they cried out, "God save me!"

The presence of God was a reality to many people who had never before felt his presence.

The convicting power of the Holy Spirit was upon

many marriages . . . then,

As suddenly as it had appeared, the dove disappeared!

It was instantly replaced by a white dove.

I told the audience the dove "like as of fire" had disappeared and had been replaced by a white one, and waited for another message from God because I didn't understand this at all.

God gave Charles the message this time and he said, "I have sent my white dove as a symbol of purification. Your marriages have been cleansed and purified. Keep them that way!"

The white dove was gone!

Hundreds of people accepted Jesus as a result of this awe-inspiring moment and many were baptized in the Holy Spirit and healed at the same time. It was estimated that around 1,800 people fell under the power of God this one night.

We may never again stand in the Shekinah glory of God until we get to heaven, but our lives will never be the same again as a result of this night.

Some people might not believe it; maybe you won't, but we have to, because we were there!

An IMPOSSIBLE MIRACLE, but it happened!

These are the days when the fire from heaven is being poured out! Oh for that day when liquid fire will come forth from the hands of ALL Spirit-filled believers! Miracles are happening, the Holy Spirit is giving visions, and the multitudes are rising up to bring glory to God! This is you — and this is me! Let us catch the vision afresh and anew!

Some people say **CHARLES** and **FRANCES HUNTER** are most noted for

...their **MIRACLE MINISTRY**.

...their ministry in the **BAPTISM WITH THE HOLY SPIRIT**.

...their ministry of teaching at their School of Ministry at the City of Light.

...The books which they write which have changed millions of lives.

...the moving of the Holy Spirit on their TV appearances.

However you feel about them, there's someone who will agree with you.

They have built the **CITY OF LIGHT CHRISTIAN CENTER** in Kingwood, Texas, a suburb of Houston, which houses a church, a school of ministry, a video school of ministry (a layman Bible school you can have in your own home), a publishing company and their office complex.

You may contact Charles and Frances Hunter by writing to them at the

CITY OF LIGHT CHRISTIAN CENTER
201 McClellan   Kingwood, TX 77339.